SoJourn to

HONDURAS

SoJourn to

HEALING

SoJourn to

HONDURAS

SoJourn to

HEALING

Why An Herbalist's View Matters
More Today Than Ever Before

BEVERLY OLIVER

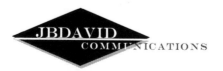

Cover Assistance by Adrienne Hailstorks

ISBN 978-0692322420

Library of Congress Control Number: 2010914687

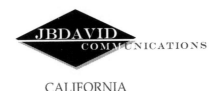

CALIFORNIA

ACKNOWLEDGMENTS

The story had to go beyond questions and answers. Readers wanted more. More clarification. More substantiation. More prose in a story that deserved it. I obliged by revamping *Seven Days in Usha Village: A Conversation With Dr. Sebi*. And even though you're about to read her transformation in the following 207 pages, independence and interdependence flow through her veins in both books.

In *Seven Days in Usha Village: A Conversation With Dr. Sebi*, laboratory reports of cured AIDS patients fill six pages. You won't find them in this book, *Sojourn to Honduras Sojourn to Healing*. You'll find recipes, a food guide and an acid and alkaline food chart in *Sojourn to Honduras*. They're absent in *Seven Days*.

Interdependence is found in the wisdom of her main subject, herbalist and nature lover Dr. Sebi. And I thank him for his approval of *Sojourn's* birth.

I thank those who wanted more and asked for more, my readers and editorial advisors Patrice Bess, Wanda Thomas, Addie Wilson-Hailstorks, Michele DeFilippo and Curtis Crutchfield. Adrienne Hailstorks' cover assistance exceeded my expectations tenfold.

I'm grateful for all the support and suspect I'll take the journey again.

Beverly Oliver

CONTENTS

INTRODUCTION   11

CHAPTER 1   PRELUDE TO HEALING   25
Acid and Alkaline Food   30

CHAPTER 2   THE INVITATION   37

CHAPTER 3   HERBALIST EMERITUS IN HONDURAS   47

CHAPTER 4   USHA VILLAGE: COSMIC, THERMAL   53
Healing Hot Spring   54
An Inner Resolve   57

CHAPTER 5   THE HEALER MAKES A CASE FOR THE
NATURAL   63
Separation From The Natural   67

CHAPTER 6   STARCH, A 400-YEAR CONSUMPTION   73
*Starch: It Gels, Swells, It Glues—Think Hardening of
the Arteries   75*

CHAPTER 7   FOOD AND THE AFRICAN GENE   83
God's Wheat, Spelt   92

CHAPTER 8   ALFREDO BOWMAN IS DR. SEBI
THE HEALER   99
Leadership   101
*Reflections on the Elderly and the Young
at Usha Village   112*
Alfredo Bowman—Ward of the State   114
They Know I Cure AIDS   118

CHAPTER 9   RELIGION GIVES WAY TO
INDEPENDENCE   123

CHAPTER 10   FREE FLOWING 133

APPENDIX   137
 Food Guide—An Introduction 137
  Fruits   141
  Vegetables   144
  Spices & Seasonings   150
  Grains   151
  Nuts & Seeds   151
  Herbal Teas   151
  Medicinal Herbs   152
 Recipes—An Introduction   155
  Breakfast   157
  Dinner   167
  Snacks   191

BIBLIOGRAPHY 199

INDEX   203

It seems evident to common reason that as nature supplies all our foods from the vegetable or herb kingdom, so should she supply all the remedies for our diseases.

–Edward E. Shook

INTRODUCTION

In 2005, retired herbalist Dr. Sebi had reached the age of 72, but I noticed the vitality of a 5-year-old at his kindergarten show and tell. On one of our daily rides around the town of La Ceiba, Honduras, he suddenly behaved in the most incredible way. I watched him leap from his truck, leave it idling in traffic, and dash his limber legs to an open field to inspect a plant that caught his eye. He examined his diamond-in-the-rough in what appeared to be widespread patches of weeds. Drivers in traffic must have been familiar with his hyperactivity. No car or truck horns blew at Dr. Sebi's sitting vehicle and passengers in waiting.

Then there was the time we were talking about his thin body, his vegetarianism and his physical strength. His high energies caught me off guard, again. With deliberate speed, he dropped his kneecaps to the stone floor of his hut without a cushion except the khaki pants he wore. When he stood up with a ballet dancer's grace and ease, I witnessed firsthand his dedication to a vegetarian's life and his calcium-rich sea moss and bladderwrack herbs. The senior citizen with knees as strong and hard as cement demonstrated unabashed compliance with his longstanding credo, "Herbs are for the healing of the nation."

Most days and evenings we talked in Dr. Sebi's large two-room round hut, a contemporary spin on a traditional African home—pale green, made of mud, and topped with a metal corrugated roof shaped like an upside down cone. It stood on the manicured mango-covered grounds of Usha Village, his healing center in Agua Caliente, a village lying at the foot of a mountain high rainforest, and about 24 miles east of La Ceiba.

His hut didn't resemble makeshift living quarters you see in television ads for saving impoverished children around the world. But it still stood simply furnished, even with the 42-inch flat screen television on the wooden stand that faced the largest piece of furniture in the hut, his king-sized bed. An African mask and two framed pictures of African art draped the walls, the lone mask, on guard it seemed, resting right above the head of the bed.

A futon with pillows and flat wood arms offered a comfortable place to sit while I listened to Dr. Sebi (SAY-BEE, ever wandering traveler). He set it across from his bed. And every morning after settling in it, my hosts served me the best cups of natural mint tea that I've ever tasted, courtesy of leaves plucked straight from bushes at Usha Village.

We talked from sunrise to sunset every day for seven days in November 2005, days when winter mornings in Honduras, Central America felt like sweltering August afternoons in New York City. Sunny or overcast, it didn't matter. The heat endured. Not long after I arrived, my hot comb straightened hair recoiled into two thick double-strand braids that I wore each day. After feeling somewhat disappointed the press didn't hold, I realized the new style suited talks of the natural in Dr. Sebi's tropical home far better than straightened tresses.

But before I get ahead of myself, let me share with you why I journeyed to Honduras and why the trip became a personal crusade to join the global food and health revolution. It's a revolution steeped in debates about GMOs, organic versus nonorganic and whether food is nutritious or comfort.

ﻬﻬﻬ

Look no farther than your dinner plate for the birthplace of disease. That's Dr. Sebi's position. What he has advocated for 30 years runs counter to organic and nonorganic food trends. Rather than recommend organic foods—some of which are starch-based and acidic—he advises a return to diets of natural, alkaline food, food that nourishes the human body, naturally energized food that prevents and minimizes the onslaught of disease. Living the first 30 years of his life with impotence, asthma and obesity, Dr. Sebi knows a thing or two about the benefits of such a change.

I felt his knowledge and contributions in the field of herbs, nutrition and natural healing deserved greater exposure. *Sojourn to Honduras, Sojourn to Healing* represents that effort, and as a springboard for understanding why Dr. Sebi's prescriptions for healing matter more today than ever before, I offer a brief sketch of my own family's experiences with diet and disease.

ಲಲಲ

I suffered with asthma between the ages of 7 and 17. For 10 years, wheezes trailed me from my home in Southeast Washington, D.C., all the way downtown to Group Health Association, my family's health care provider. But somehow I managed to sing in the junior choir at Little Ark Baptist Church.

Car rides to church, by way of the Anacostia Bridge, always sparked a rhythmical singsong. I'd sing water! water! wa-ter! while I watched waves ripple and fold against the stony edge of the Anacostia River—a fun respite from the concrete at Ketcham Elementary's playground. But crossing the river to go to the doctor, with little oxygen in my lungs to allow even the slightest whisper, I looked out the car's window and wheezed at the water below the bridge. I couldn't sing down to it and I wondered if it was as sad as I was because I couldn't. Short breaths and glassy eyes carried me over the wavelets to Group Health.

Once over the bridge, habitual nighttime rides past our country's historic landmarks diverted my attention from sickness to awe. The Potomac River shined across the Tidal Basin, while ground lights flooded the Bureau of Engraving, the Washington Monument and the White House, those colossal stones hovering above us and all a rock's throw from the clinic.

2121 Pennsylvania Avenue, Northwest. Group Health—GHA as it was identified on the rectangular green vertical sign attached to the side of the eight-story building—was practically my second home. Sometimes I arrived in my pajamas and robe, always escorted by my mother and usually by Yellow Cab, Capitol Cab, or the car of my father's best friend and co-worker Mr. Davidson. When I was old enough to take the bus alone, a task my mother insisted I learn posthaste to free up her time to take care of my baby sister Pam, the bus marked 34 Friendship Heights dropped me off at Group Health. I stepped through the revolving glass doors and landed in what must have been the most sanitized lobby on earth, a blend of alcohol and Pine Sol swirling in the air.

I found relief at Group Health, relief from sudden bouts of short breaths late at night or in the middle of the day. Most attacks struck at will in humidity-slapping summertime when air swelled with not only grass and dirt playful kids kicked up, but dog and cat dander as well. When a stray dog wandered within a few feet of me and my neighborhood playmates, I knew a trip downtown followed. I never knew exactly when my lungs would tighten. I just knew they would. I knew that like clockwork a doctor's cold stethoscope against my chest and back would confirm oxygen's struggle to enter and leave my body. Wheezes with every inhale, every exhale. Gurgling, bubbling phlegm squeezed and expanded in my chest and lungs like an accordion.

With some anxiety about these persistent attacks, hers and mine, my mother drilled me to cough up the gunk. "Cough it up. Cough it up and spit it out," she'd race to tell me. I tried. Tried hard every time and every time a wad of slime slid back deeper in my chest.

As I think back on those days, I was spitting out thick saliva in my mouth instead of pulling the mucous from deep down in my chest, as deep as my diaphragm. If my mother had advised me to pull from there, like our choir director when she instructed us to pull air from that deep place, I'm sure I would have had more success pulling up and spitting out "the gunk." Ma, if you're reading this from Heaven, you probably should have said, "Hawk it. Hawk it up Beverly Ann. Hawk it up from the depths of your soul."

I received shots to help clear my lungs, as well as over-the-counter pills Primatene and Tedral, well-known and used asthma medications in the 1970s. They cleared my lungs like the hot coffee my mother used to give me, but just like the coffee, they kept me awake at night, and the wheezing always returned. Why didn't I use an inhaler? I never could coordinate inhaling with squirting medicine down my lungs, even after repeated instructions from my mother—her asthma more severe than mine, aggravated by a half a pack of Winston cigarettes she smoked every day.

By the time I was a junior in high school, I was on a weekly regimen of shots to desensitize my allergies. I must admit they helped. Allergic reactions to cats, dogs, ragweed, pollen and all other substances that bring asthmatics down ended—all except one.

If you know anything about southern cooking in the United States, you know it's starch-rich and creamy: black-eyed peas, cornbread, biscuits and gravy, white rice, grits, potatoes, macaroni and cheese. I love this food. Ate lots of it growing up in D.C., a tableful on Sundays, Thanksgiving, Christmas, and Easter, cooked by southern parents and relatives from Orangeburg County, South Carolina.

On a typical Oliver plate you'd find fried pork chops, collard greens seasoned with cured ham, rice or mashed potatoes with brown gravy and onions, potato salad, biscuits and a nice cold glass of sweet ice tea. We'd expect candied yams for Thanksgiving, but my mother's sweet potato pie made rounds at the table as a regular Sunday dessert. Friday, my favorite meal day, was a fish fry kind of day: salmon cakes or my mother's favorite fish, croakers. Grits, oozing with butter on my plate, or fried potatoes and onions, rounded it all out.

I ate that way as a student at Howard University too, not as much as I did as a child but I never turned it down when friends suggested we eat lunch at an off-campus grill—a quick-cooking fried chicken leg and French fries the first choice. And while at Howard, just a few years after all those shots, I noticed an all too familiar shortness of breath. No one informed us soul food eaters that every bite, every down home morsel, ushered in far-reaching health complications.

MY BELOVED FRANCES

I have a black and white photograph of my godmother Frances, taken when she was somewhere around 18 years old. At first glance, she's a polished, dapper Negro woman of the early 1940s; her hair cropped short, and pressed and curled the Madam C. J. Walker way. A white blouse with pearl buttons and a dark business suit cover her poised body. The jacket fits straight and wide on her shoulders and narrows down and inward at her waist. Only the top half of her body appears in the center of the picture, revealing a slender woman. I'd guess 110 to 115 pounds.

Well beyond slender by the time I was born (I'm a baby boomer), Frances, at 5'2, had grown stout around her midriff and wore a C-cup bra. I never knew her exact weight, but thinking back to the 1970s I'd say she weighed between 150 and 160 pounds. Every pound followed by her ever present coifed femininity. It followed her everywhere: cotton lounge dresses at home, some plaid, others pastel stripes. In public, dresses and skirt sets even when pantsuits were in vogue. Clearly a captain's mate on fishing trips with my godfather Leroy, she wore crisp khaki pants and spotless Decks tennis shoes.

Frances and her family the McDowells moved from South Carolina to Washington, D.C. during the Great Migration, that period in U.S. history between 1910 and 1960 when over 5 million Negroes moved from post-slavery southern towns to northern cities—their southern cooking in tow.

Besides my mother, Frances reigned supreme as the best southern cook I ever knew. Lest I forget, Sylvia Woods of Sylvia's Restaurant in Harlem, New York ranks high in that league. She's another South Carolina daughter.

Frances' Sunday meals included delicious Crisco-laden southern fare, including her homemade biscuits and what I considered a strange part of the cow to eat—cow's tongue. Sometimes I flinched my nose at it while it cooled in a big pot on the stove. Frances caught me one Sunday and brushed me away. "Go on away from here. That's for Leroy," she'd say.

And he loved it. Smiled at me across the dining room table when he ate it. So one Sunday I decided to give it a try, just a little taste of the thick eight-inch slab of pink meat.

Leroy carved a piece for me and laid it on my plate. I stared at it, wondering if I should douse it with butter or gravy. I decided against both. I cut a small piece from the slice, chewed, swallowed and smiled back at Leroy. Cow's tongue tasted just like ham.

Baked goods? My mouth waters thinking about Frances' German chocolate cake. Truly a great southern cook. But my beloved lady, unfortunately, lived with high blood pressure.

She never mentioned it, never complained. She swallowed her medication every day and cooked the foods she knew best, the way she knew best, as do all cooks of starch-rich, creamy foods. I never heard it from her if her pressure rose too high and made her feel bad. Leroy, always quiet and composed, passed the news along to us, including the news one night in 1979, that Frances had stopped taking her medicine and died that evening. Frances loved me and cared for me like the child she never bore. I loved her too.

Twenty years after she died, Leroy drove up from Washington to visit me in New York. Frances and her health, never far from our lips, dominated the conversations. Leroy often repeated stories about her, especially the time they decided to buy and sleep in twin beds because Frances didn't want to be intimate anymore.

I was an adult. I had an understanding of life then that I didn't have when Frances lived, so I defended her. Her decision laid deep-rooted in some incident in her life, I thought. I knew she cared for Leroy too much to sleep in a separate bed and deny him intimacy. What went wrong? Was her medication making her sick? Was she working too hard? Frances had been a housekeeper and cook for a Kennedy administration lawyer in D.C., and with Leroy, operated an office maintenance service in the evening. I rallied Frances' cause but Leroy subdued me when he said doctors found tumors in her uterus the size of grapefruits. When they removed them Frances changed and decided she didn't want to have sex anymore. I was sad for her and Leroy. I thought the tumors not only prevented them from having children but may have caused her high blood pressure. I asked Leroy if Frances saw a therapist or counselor after her surgery. He said no.

Leroy had his health issues too, his Vick's nasal spray a constant companion. Without fail he sprayed it up his nostrils to relieve his sinusitis. In conversations after dinner, he'd spray into each nostril. We'd watch football games—the Washington Redskins our favorite—and he'd spray it. After Frances died his blood pressure rose too. We all loved each other and we ate well, quantitatively speaking.

ৰৰৰ

Could it be that in my family's story you saw your own? A father or husband with an incessant snore due to a clogged nasal passage. A mother or sister battling fibroid tumors. A friend's three-day connection to a dialysis machine, or maybe your own daily shot of insulin.

My mother and my godparents Frances and Leroy passed on before I could share with them the source of their health problems. While it may be too late for them or your late relatives and friends, healing stands at the threshold for those of us willing to look squarely in the face of disease and diet and see that life-sustaining changes are not only needed, but have a solution in place to meet the needs. And you'll find planted deep within its foundation, deep within the recesses of healing, an herbalist called Dr. Sebi. I met him long before my journey to Honduras. I met him in my hometown Washington, D.C.

It's time to move past the debate of alternative medicine versus traditional medicine, and to focus on what works, what doesn't, for whom, and under which circumstances.

–Deepak Chopra

Chapter 1

Prelude to Healing

Dr. Sebi's lecture circuit, in full swing in the early 1980s, included stops in several mid-Atlantic urban cities. I sat in on one of his lectures when he stopped in Washington, D.C. sometime around 1982 or '83. With an instructor's stance right at the beginning he announced, "The herbs are for the healing of the nation."

That evening he stood slender and statuesque at the Community Warehouse, a food co-op and lecture space in Northeast Washington. He looked more like a Maasai tribesman than a Honduran in Central America. He was born there in 1933 in the mountainous and tropical village of Ilanga, Honduras. By the time he reached Washington, D.C., he had already lived and worked in the United States for over 30 years, married, and fathered seven children, and with dedicated patronage from niche followers, used his herbal compounds to cure clients suffering from all manner of disease, including cancer, diabetes, lupus and sickle cell anemia.

I didn't know any of this or his birth name, Alfredo Bowman, when I saw him that first time. My reason for going to hear his lecture was twofold: I was in the early stages of endometriosis and felt uneasy about having the recommended laparoscopy. My gynecologist forecasted an incision below my navel and a small fiber optic telescope inserted in that incision browsing my uterus to locate the problem. I was pretty apprehensive about this surgical and minimally invasive procedure. So John Davies, a vegetarian colleague of mine at WHUR-FM, suggested that I not only consult Dr. Sebi (self-moniker), but share his advice in a radio show about natural healing.

The longer I listened to Dr. Sebi that night, listened to him clear up misperceptions, life-threatening misperceptions, people have accepted about food and diseases for generations, I realized John had turned me on to a good idea. It was the first time I had ever heard someone get to the root of bad health.

ৡৡৡ

Dr. Sebi's Spanish accent didn't prevent him from speaking clear and robust English. His delivery and determined persona reminded me of the late stage and film actor Yul Brynner, when he played the willful King of Siam in the film *The King and I*.

Along with the history of food, Dr. Sebi stood before us and touted the supremacy of a vegetarian's life, but cautioned his audience that what appears to be and what has been traditionally called nutritious vegetables, are acid-based stimulants. Now, if there's any reaction that has influenced Dr. Sebi's relationship with his public over the past 30 years, it is without a doubt the rejection of his comments about what is food and what is not, especially carrots and garlic.

"They're hybrids. Both will undermine your immune system," he claimed and has claimed for years.

The carrot, a hybrid? That garden variety made orange by Dutch geneticists in the 17th century, and the one we eat today, yes. The first carrot, a wild carrot, no.

Wild carrots now and over 2,000 years ago are white, purple and yellow. They were used by ancient Greeks and Romans for medicinal purposes according to the California Foundation for Agriculture. They have a woody texture and bitter taste. But selective breeding down through the years changed all that. Plant geneticists inserted large amounts of beta-carotene in the parent plant, giving wild carrots a sweet taste and the familiar orange color.

It is this breeding, this change in the composition of a natural plant into something other than its natural state that drives Dr. Sebi's rejection of hybrids, especially hybrids passed onto human diets.

కళకళకళ

His words pulsated throughout the room. No microphone or bull horn needed for the room full of Black Americans from varied lifestyles. Black Americans, it still has a resounding ring to it. By 1982, we had shed the fight word "black" of the 1950s and early 60s and embraced "Black American," a holdover from James Brown's soulful admonition and hit R&B record, *Say it Loud, I'm Black and I'm Proud.*

Women at Dr. Sebi's presentation wore hairstyles reflecting the pride: afros, precise lines of cornrows, while others wore trendy sculptured braids. A few had perms. Businessmen and college students sat in, with smells of frankincense and myrrh oil spreading around all of us.

He scanned a sea of interested alert faces and spoke to us as if his passion for herbs and his knowledge of natural foods equaled ours, as if we were his partner on the journey to right health and right eating. But when he uttered the words acid and alkaline food, we responded with blank stares. Acid? Was he speaking of carbonated sodas? Alkaline? The same stares continued when he mentioned pH. It was my first time hearing it.

Twenty years would pass before I understood the necessity of knowing these terms and making one of them, alkaline food, a staple in my kitchen. The one word I'd use to describe this newfound knowledge is treasure. My disclaimer is, however, I am not an herbalist, nutritionist, doctor or scientist but a seeker, an inquirer, and after all I've been through with asthma, a lover of good health and delicious healthy food.

ھ ھ ھ

Despite Dr. Sebi's own Afrocentric look—a cotton dashiki top and loose cotton pants—some in the audience sat surprised by his comments, especially his comparisons of natural and hybrid foods. Whispers of doubt filled the room. But he convinced me a larger audience—generations of diabetics and asthmatics, generations of the hypertensive and the obese—should hear what he had to say about health and nutrition. I invited him to WHUR to speak in a four-part radio series on herbs and natural healing.

We recorded a session a little over an hour, and as I think back, once alone in the studio with the taped interview, I soon realized a difficult edit lay ahead. You just can't put it all in the program, no matter how great or informative. The final cut yielded four 10-minute shows with theme music by composer and piano player Lonnie Liston Smith. His jazz fusion and the mellifluous vocals of his brother Donald rendered a serene cosmic aesthetic to each show and complemented Dr. Sebi's rare gentle voicing of the cosmic procession of life. WHUR broadcast the series in the weekly newsmagazine *The Sunday Digest*.

Now, 26 years later, rising health care costs in the United States, little or no health care in developing countries, more challenging diseases reported every day, assurances of organic and nonorganic food choices when a more appropriate focus should be the consumption of natural alkaline foods, are all evidence that an herbalist's view is still a good listen. A journey to Honduras, Central America in November 2005 not only shined a light on Dr. Sebi's background and long-held views, it led to a firsthand look at a public willing to feel better and eat better, but lacking sufficient exposure to information about healing and food.

I'm reminded of a Saturday afternoon I stopped by Dr. Sebi's office in Los Angeles after that first trip to Usha

Village. His staff had compiled a cookbook with vegetarian recipes, a cookbook chock full of meals they'd been working on for some time but sat unpublished. They gave me a copy and from that I printed more and dropped them off at his office, considering it the best I could do at that moment to help others eat proper foods.

Clients flowed in and out of the office buying Dr. Sebi's herbal products and the Saturday afternoon meal of the day, vegetarian lasagna, a succulent dish made so by Dr. Sebi's daughter Xave.

A slender African American woman who appeared to be in her mid-40s waited with her 4-year-old daughter to buy the lunch and an herbal shake. When she heard me talk to the staff about the cookbook, she gave a frantic search deep down in her shoulder bag for a piece of paper to write down some of the recipes. When I noticed the paper she pulled out looked like a bill of some sort, folded and too small for the simplest recipe, I knew the cookbook and a story about an herbalist from Honduras were long overdue. I gave the lady my draft copy of the cookbook.

Acid and Alkaline Food

ৡৢৡৢৡৢ

Organic Food? Inorganic Food? But is it Acid or
Alkaline? Is it Natural?

So what were those words Dr. Sebi mentioned—hybrids, acid, alkaline—and what did they have to do with the asthma that seemed to rear its ahead again and again after all my eternal visits to the allergist at Group Health? After 20 years of hearing them, my journey led me on a search for all things acid and alkaline. For instance,

pH = potential for Hydrogen, a measurement of acidity or alkalinity; a measurement of the concentration of hydrogen ions in a substance. The pH scale of food and human blood runs from 0 to 14.

The lower the number on the pH scale, the more acidic the food, food that breaks down the body's protective mucous membrane. Acidosis is a common occurrence. Sinusitis is another. Starch-based and refined foods are moderately to highly acidic (beans, flour, sugar, rice, eggs, milk, cheese, cassava, potatoes).

ACID   ALKALINE (natural)

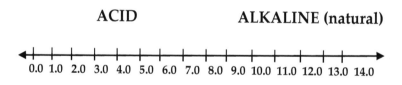

0.0 1.0 2.0 3.0 4.0 5.0 6.0 7.0 8.0 9.0 10.0 11.0 12.0 13.0 14.0

pH Scale

The higher the number on the pH scale, the more alkaline the food, food that nourishes the body and allows blood and oxygen to flow freely. Alkaline food supports the immune system. Examples of alkaline foods are green vegetables, chickpeas, most fruits, maple sugar and syrup, mushrooms, onions, almonds. The pH value of healthy human blood is 7.365. Take a look at a table of acid and alkaline food.

ACID/ALKALINE FOOD CHART

ACID FOODS	ALKALINE FOODS
Tend to Weaken/Clog Body's Cells and Immune System (Oxygen flow hampered) (Blood flow hampered)	Tend to Strengthen Body's Cells and Immune System (Oxygen flows freely) (Blood flows freely)
pH range is 0 to 6.9	pH range is 7.0 to 14.0
Cow's Milk	Almond Milk
Corn Puffs	Kamut Puffs
Sugar, Artificial Sugar	Maple Sugar, Maple Syrup
Salt	Sea Salt, Onion Sea Salt
Black Pepper	Cayenne Pepper
Potatoes	Chickpeas
Yogurt	Apple Sauce
Meat	Mushrooms

ACID/ALKALINE FOOD CHART

ACID FOODS	ALKALINE FOODS
Tend to Weaken/Clog Body's Cells and Immune System (Oxygen flow hampered) (Blood flow hampered)	Tend to Strengthen Body's Cells and Immune System (Oxygen flows freely) (Blood flows freely)
pH range is 0 to 6.9	pH range is 7.0 to 14.0
Bread	Spelt Bread
Bleached/Unbleached Flour	Spelt Flour, Chickpea Flour
Peanuts/Peanut Butter	Almonds/Almond Butter
Navy, Pinto and Lima Beans, Peas	Green Beans, Leafy Green Vegetables
White Rice	Wild Rice
Pasta, Noodles, Spaghetti	Spelt Elbow Macaroni, Spelt Pasta, Spelt Spaghetti
Butter	Olive Oil

Awakening is the foundation of every
kind of change.

–Thich Nhat Hanh

CHAPTER 2

THE INVITATION

I relocated to Los Angeles in December 2003 and planned to flex my creativity in drama and writing, even though I embraced the idea that someday I'd work on another *Wade in the Water: African American Sacred Music Traditions*. That Peabody award-winning radio documentary embodied ideals and prowess of good leadership I've admired for an eternity. It was an honor to be its Production Assistant.

About 18 months after I arrived in L.A. I ran out of my Eva Salve, one of Dr. Sebi's products for females. I'd been using it since the 1980s, rubbing it on my pelvic area whenever I felt cysts rising. The pale yellow ointment furrows deep beneath the skin, wrapping intrusive tissue, those solid balls of mucous that creep in, attaching themselves to weak unprotected pockets in the body. Eva Salve dissolves the mass in a matter of hours it seems. I find, too, that when the pungent sulfuric smell bursts from its uncapped container and rises high in the nostrils, the most stubborn packed phlegm clears a path. I vowed never to be without that most treasured natural product.

I ordered it from Dr. Sebi's first and now former Miami-based company, The Fig Tree. When I called about a new order the operator informed an office in Los Angeles sold the salve and that I could pick it up there. It belonged to Dr. Sebi and I wasted no time going. I arrived on his office doorstep less than a week later in late August 2005.

That afternoon visit marked a new phase in my acquaintance with Dr. Sebi. The extent of our meetings in the 80s rarely amounted to more than my attendance at his lectures and the radio station interview. Business filled every minute, no time for small talk. I expected to keep that pace—say hello, let him know I lived in Los Angeles, buy the Eva Salve and leave.

ॐ ॐ ॐ

A buzzer unlocked the front door of a lime green two-story building that housed Dr. Sebi's Office, LLC on the lower level. A slender attractive woman with a short gray Afro appeared from behind curtains of a back office. She managed Dr. Sebi's company and called herself Matun (MA-TUNE). Her height appeared to be five feet four or five and she wore a sleeveless black A-line dress that looked more cocktail than office attire.

I found her quiet and a bit distant as she walked over to the glass showcase of herbal products.

"I'm here to pick up some Eva Salve," I said, somewhat anxious to get pass the sale and onto a visit with Dr. Sebi.

"Is Dr. Sebi here?"

Her steady eyes met mine and she said, "He's not here at the moment."

I suspected curious spectators mingled with the sincere in Dr. Sebi's line of business so I quickly introduced myself not only as a longtime patron of Dr. Sebi's products, but as someone who interviewed him years ago. That broke the ice.

With her Caribbean accent she told me Dr. Sebi was living in Honduras, Central America. She asked for my phone number and said she would pass it and my greetings to Dr. Sebi. I accepted that and decided not to take up a lot of her time with the thrill of my presence in Dr. Sebi's space. Before I left with the salve I looked around, and in the browse I faced a three feet by four feet painting on an easel. I viewed a pensive man with short white hair and a white goatee—a fitting impression of an elder Dr. Sebi.

Nearly three weeks went by. Then out of the blue, when the thrill of occupying his space passed, a voice on the other end of my cell phone said, "Beverly, this is Sebi." Was it Dr. Sebi? It sounded like him. I was almost sure it was. We never talked on the phone in the past because appointments and phone calls were handled by his assistants.

"How are you?" I asked.

"Not as good as you."

Yes, it was him, calling from Los Angeles. And just as I charged to his company to pick up the salve, I rushed back, this time, to his suite on the upper level of his building.

Matun greeted me again and led me upstairs to Dr. Sebi. The sun poured through a skylight to light the whole top floor, including a small foyer furnished with large thick floor pillows and two chairs. He welcomed me there, tall, upright, just as he stood 20 years earlier in Washington, D.C. His voice the same as well, devoid of any sign of aging. His lifestyle, for the most part unchanged, differed in a minor way to him, in a significant way to me—he retired from healing and counseling.

I went to visit him in peace but instead I received an unexpected jolt. Few lectures. No more client consultations. Who on earth, I asked, will pick up the torch and carry on a much needed business?

"My daughter Xave is running the business," he announced proud and emphatic. "She can mix herbs 10 times better than me."

My joy evaporated into the herbal air. I felt I'd lost a trusted doctor when he announced his retirement. He assured me his company remained in reliable hands. "That salve you bought? Xave made that batch."

I wanted him to leave something behind besides a company that bore his name. I asked him why he hadn't written a book, a nightstand reference we could all turn to in his absence. Within seconds of asking the question, he pulled out a manuscript of 140 pages—his life story. He called it *The Cure: The Autobiography of Dr. Sebi "Mama Hay"* and shared it with me in a review copy. I read it and learned things about him that never surfaced 20 years before: He travelled the seas as a young merchant seaman before settling in North America; Martin Luther King, Jr. Hospital employee Alfredo Bowman, steam engineer, becomes Dr. Sebi the herbalist and treats more than a few celebrated personalities. When I offered editorial suggestions for his book, he offered me a plane ticket to his native home, Honduras.

వ్యూమ్మ

Sunday, November 6, 2005. My flight plans from Los Angeles International Airport to La Ceiba, Honduras included seats on three planes operated by TACA Airlines, a Latin American carrier serving North, South and Central America and the Caribbean. Lines at check-in snaked around with Spanish-speaking travelers, a midnight departure no bother. Babies cooed. Sleepy toddlers cried. Some held tight to strollers. Men with shiny black hair slid thick, elephant-sized bulges of luggage across the counter. I saw a few Caucasian-looking passengers, no African Americans. They could have been there. I was awed by this new international experience, preoccupied with my own presence in a sea of Latin Americans. Everyone spoke Spanish except me. My Spanish interpreter and the sponsor of my trip waited for me on the other end. Dr. Sebi assured me I'd be fine travelling with TACA.

After five hours and two stops, one in San Salvador, El Salvador, and another in San Pedro Sula, we landed in La Ceiba, Honduras.

Without regalia or suit and tie, Dr. Sebi carried his usual diplomat's stance in the terminal, even in his brown sandals, white short sleeved cotton shirt and matching white loose fitting cotton pants. He stood beside Matun smiling with his eyes. I found him receptive, his hug firm, not a hint of a healer's roadblocks down through the years or his own past ill health.

When cab drivers vied for his attention, he greeted them but one pre-selected comrade stood ready to take my suitcase and drive us to Agua Caliente, a town 24 miles east of La Ceiba. Agua Caliente, Spanish for "hot water" and the location of Dr. Sebi's hot spring and 20-year-old healing center, Usha Village.

The cab travelled on a two-lane paved road, a blacktop that cut straight through miles of low lying flora, palm trees, and scattered one-story adobe houses. Children looked out of glassless windows. I watched thin mutts mosey along in yards and beside the road. We drove past new housing development construction in limbo. Then, within seconds, the next frame in the cab's moving picture revealed a billboard that offered comfort and luxury at completed houses.

I learned that more than luxury Dr. Sebi prefers peace and life as close to nature as possible. Almond trees and mango trees flourished at Usha Village. My nighttime snack included three juicy fibrous mangoes I gathered each day. They had fallen from trees that stood on 20 acres, property replete with a paved entrance stretching about one eighth of a mile long from the main gate up to the first cabin.

The cabins—Dr. Sebi calls them huts—are one-story, one-room structures with a twin bed, some with a double, a nightstand holding an oscillating table fan, a chair, and a wooden wardrobe. The tiled bathroom has a bathtub with sides that stand about three feet high, which I found a tad unsettling to climb over the first time since I'm a little more than two feet higher than the top of it. But once I settled underneath the shower I found a soothing gem: natural thermal water.

శ్రీశ్రీశ్రీ

By the time I got out of bed each morning, Dr. Sebi and Matun had been awake and talking with Usha Village staff and groundskeepers for three hours. I intended to wake up early too, especially after Dr. Sebi informed me the first day I arrived he usually ended his days around six o'clock in the evening and rose before the sun—a custom since the days he lived with his grandmother.

Whenever I sleep in the tropics, my mind takes a habitual switch to summer vacation—tranquility, rest, mid-morning casual risings. But on Monday morning, it had been just a few weeks since Hurricane Beta paid Central America a visit, and Gamma was thrashing her way west from the Caribbean Sea. None of this crossed my mind. The sun rose. It set. Sparse clouds hovered above the village. By the third day in Honduras though, 80-degree temperatures by nine in the morning made it clear to me a casual walk from my cabin to Dr. Sebi's hut a few yards away would end in a cotton blouse sticking to my skin. Dr. Sebi's cooled hut offered relief, and before I left Honduras I was waking up about an hour after daybreak.

At night, before or after a warm rainfall, frog calls filled the village. This nightly performance in the bush, an unseen but heard symphony, swelled with resonant harmonious frog croaks that must have come from the lungs of creatures large and small. One evening, after a talk with Dr. Sebi, one of the palm-size chanters greeted me at the door of my cabin.

The only true science of medicine is the intelligent use of nature's only real medicinal remedies—herbs.

–Edward E. Shook

1

CHAPTER 3

HERBALIST EMERITUS IN HONDURAS

Torrential rain fell Thursday night in Honduras, as it had since my arrival on Sunday. In cycles it splashed against the cabin waking me then lulling me back to sleep with a steady rhythmical fall. All the trees of Usha Village—palm, mango, almond—swayed and clapped in the torrent. When I stepped outside my cabin every morning, I noticed only a few fallen palm leaves and slim branches had left traces of the downpour. Heat had assisted the rain in its disappearing act. And just as it has across Earth, global warming has knocked on Central America's door, changing the air of Dr. Sebi's boyhood tropics. *"There is less moisture in the air than when I was a child,"* he informed me. *"Because right here in the little village of Jutiapa it used to be cold, cold, cold where I had to wear a sweater and you couldn't see five feet in front of you. The fog was so thick. Now, there's no fog and it's warm because they cut the trees down. But basically, you still have the moisture, the fauna, the flora that one expects to exist in a tropical country. And I guess I enjoy that."*

ॐॐॐ

He lounged on one of those warm Honduran evenings, resting his t-shirt clad upper torso on mounds of pillows that pressed against a wood headboard. His brown six-foot-three frame stretched out long on the bed he used like a reclining chair. And from this reposed, carefree posture he regressed, re-lived, and lambasted. He shared tales of global adventures and those of debate-filled confrontations over herbs, health and food.

"Any grain that is made—corn, wheat, rice—these things are starch. Starch is not a food. Starch is a chemical. Starch is what you use to separate region. I did because I'm an engineer. I understand how to use starch. Starch is not a food."

He either reclined or sat on the edge of his bed touching his thick white goatee with quick gorilla scratches while he raved the naysayers who opposed and questioned his sandal-wearing lifestyle and mentality. He recounted details about Caribbean, African and American travels and travails: suspicions of quackery in St. Croix, restoring movement to a paralysis patient in St. Martin, curing a young girl of sickle cell anemia in Washington, D.C. Then there was the rattling off of impotence statistics (high and rising higher in developing countries); infants born with diabetes were just as deplorable to him. It was an awakening I hadn't expected on that trip, and looking in his eyes, it was obvious the memories were an unsettling experience for him.

One night, I sat stoic as Dr. Sebi, with a father's chastisement, recited how the journey from abundance to poverty has left Africa lacking proper decisions about health and nutrition.

"Since we find that the African people are starving because the corn suffered a drought or the wheat, well, that's okay. Let us understand, was the corn really nourishing our body? The answer is no. It was stimulating our body, not nourishing."

I knew his humanity ran deeper than his incisive criticisms, so I asked him how to change the global state of health and nutrition. I asked even though I noticed throughout our talks his indiscreet confessions and opinions were easier to come by than his advice. Reflective, steadfast, stubborn almost, he looked me straight in the eye several times and said things are not going to change, especially if the diet hasn't changed.

That mood and venting flowed in and out of our talks that week. So, too, did his Honduran staff and groundskeepers, several of Mayan Indian descent. Those minor interruptions to tend to village matters subdued Dr. Sebi and softened the recollection of a 25-year, oftentimes rocky journey with healing, health and food.

Urgent, prophetic and without remorse, he spoke to me about past and present states of health and food. He disclosed personal and political events that included friendship with 1960s activist and civic leader Stokely Carmichael.

"I met Stokely Carmichael many, many years ago in New York. He came to me and I gave him the compounds. He began to do well but he had to return to fight the revolution. And the food

that revolutionary people eat is always hogs, starches and some uric acid."

He recounted his days as a friend and healer to personalities unknown and known, including Michael Jackson and hip hop singer Lisa "Left Eye" Lopes.

"Lisa knew that she was sick and that she wanted to be healed and that she wanted to get away from that place that she was in. And she did it."

Memories of an alienating time in Zimbabwe stirred up some unrest. When we talked about the state of health in Zimbabwe and other African countries he commented, *"They're eating stimulants. They are not nourishing their bodies."* More about Zimbabwe in Chapter 8.

The cushy futon I sat on, along with the rest of the front of the hut, transformed into a makeshift recording studio. I used a Marantz cassette recorder and an Electro Voice microphone to record a week-long conversation with Dr. Sebi, herbalist emeritus. He obliged without hesitation, ready to have his say, ready to collaborate and expand details of his future autobiography.

My sojourn to Honduras allowed us to trek the globe together, a relationship far more substantial than our first encounter in Washington, D.C.

Improving dietary habit is a societal,
not just an individual problem.
Therefore, it demands a population-based,
multi-sectoral, multi-disciplinary,
and culturally relevant approach.

**World Health Organization,
"Global Strategy on Diet, Physical
Activity and Health."
April 19, 2004**

CHAPTER 4

USHA VILLAGE: COSMIC, THERMAL

The fan circulated a chill that made the hut a comfortable place to drink hot mint tea Matun brewed every morning. A shot of Dr. Sebi's sea moss elixir followed—an acquired taste, but an excellent source of calcium and iron.

I sipped and Matun tidied up an already neat hut, with the exception of a rug slightly out of place and a large bath towel on the futon. She changed the linen on Dr. Sebi's lounge-bed-turned-podium while he bathed, and listened with me as the bathtub transformed into Dr. Sebi's lecture space too.

I had a feeling I was an engaged objective listener he hadn't hosted in a long time. And for me, it had been weeks since I heard this kind of mental stimulation and I appreciated the opportunity. The hut filled with a string of his insights that only my tape recorder could capture with accuracy, but there was enough of a pause for me to ask what led to his conclusions about food and health. More than once, with respect one gives a king or queen, he pointed to the cosmic arrangement of life. He never used the word instinct or intuition or spiritual, only cosmic arrangement.

"It's an energy that you receive," he said. *"It's not a piece of thing or stuff you put on a blackboard. It's an energy that gives you the privilege to act on that which is necessary to preserve your life. That is the connection. What is it? Well I have to use some English words, right? Well, there aren't any English words to describe that. Because life was here long before there was an English word. So we can't use an English word to describe that. Food begins to show us a whole lot of things. Nobody came to tell us that we could not eat rice and beans and that we shouldn't put blood in our mouth. Nobody came with that message. But we found it. So how did we get the message? There again, the same way the eagle got its message to make a nest, the cosmic arrangement of things, from the vibration."*

Healing Hot Spring

ॐॐॐ

He arranged a thermal water bath for me in one of the bathhouses he built behind the cabins. It was a short walk, just a few yards away at the bottom of a grassy hill. A groundskeeper prepared the bath by opening the tap to let water pour in from the hot spring, a phenomenal body of water I'd experienced only in books and television. In 30 minutes, water filled a bathtub large enough to hold at least three people. Alone, I dunked in and out of what felt like the

54

smoothest water that ever touched my body. I waded in it for the full 20 minutes Dr. Sebi recommended. Euphoria covered me 10 minutes in and stayed with me while I walked back up the hill to my cabin. My mind filled with images of an African village near the Congo River, a lush, bountiful habitat 1,000 years ago. I cringed when Dr. Sebi informed me he might sell Usha Village.

I dressed and went back to his hut for another round of talks. I told him he had a gold mine in his thermal water, his own natural heat pump supplying all that smooth phenomenal comfort. Humbled and not surprised, he explained my reaction.

"Everybody who comes here they're amazed. They come here with Kaposi's sarcoma. That's the last stage of AIDS, when the sores are on your skin, breaking down your first defense, your skin. They go into the thermal baths and in four days the sores have disappeared as if they were never there. A man came here from Argentina with lung cancer. But instead of him going in the bath water, I put him in the sauna where he is now going to inhale the waters and vapors into his lungs. In two months his lung cancer disappeared completely. So now, why does it have such a calming effect on the body that when you lay in it you go ah-h-h, this is so delicious? It goes to the pores, the high concentration of sulfur, phosphorous and iron. Sulfur is the main ingredient in thermal waters. And sulfur, natural sulfur, because there is such a thing as artificial sulfur. That's the one you give those cows in the barns. Natural sulfur, organic sulfur, is the greatest thing for your lungs. The cells of the lungs are made of sulfur. Like the bones are made of calcium. The blood is iron. Sulfur begins to do repairs in the lungs. Phosphorous is great company for iron, which is going

to electrify you and at the same time have a calming effect. The pH of thermal waters is 8, 9.6, 8.9, which is extremely high. Any substance that has such a high concentration of hydrogen, iron concentration, it is effective in healing because it is oxygen that heals."

It was a good marriage I thought, his integration of thermal dynamics and his love of herbs. He had morphed from Alfredo Bowman steam engineer to Dr. Sebi the healer.

"A steam engineer is an individual that understands the science of thermal dynamics, which is heat exchange," he said. "I was a steam engineer and I learned from the pH balance of things how to maintain the water. How could you transpose that into healing? Well yes, because I have to maintain a pH balance of 6.9, which is slightly on the acid side of life. So I concluded that if 6.9 is acid and 7.1 is alkaline, well all the herbs that heal should be on the alkaline side. But when I began to look at the menus of all the healers in America, they had peppermint — acid. They had aloe vera — acid. They had echinacea — acid. They had don quoi — acid. Every herb that they used, with the exception of a few, like burdock and yellow dock, which are alkaline, and dandelion, the rest of them are acid. So I said well where did American healers get their menu? As I looked at their menu and I looked at the European menu, it is the same. I said oh my God, something is wrong with this picture because they are both in error. But how would they examine what Europe says is true? You don't have any other perspective to put it against to say oh no, this cannot work because I have this as an example. You have no example. I had nature's way. So when I was presented with the mechanical way of treating disease I could see the difference because I had the natural way. With the natural way it becomes a barometer. I could measure the unnatural. But if you only have the unnatural, you cannot meas-

ure because that's all you have. How would you measure it? You have to have the natural to understand the unnatural."

An Inner Resolve

శ్రీశ్రీశ్రీ

Instead of picking up where I left off in the 1980s, there were moments at Usha Village when I felt I was meeting Dr. Sebi for the first time. He mauled formal education like a pit bull in a dogfight. "It prevents you from seeing life outside the box," he said without remorse.

In an afternoon conversation he sat upright on his bed stirred up, ready to prove that self-confidence, inner strength trumps education. I doused this flare up with a smile. I visualized my liberal arts training, from kindergarten through college: my music and art lessons, my language, geography and English lessons—all favorites. Anchored with that thought, yet open to what the accomplished healer had to say, I listened.

"I was given a disease that I had to address, a disease that you would never find the solution in any book. That disease is known as lockjaw. Once your jaw is locked it will remain locked and you will die. So I sat in front of her and I saw her dying and everybody was in the house, approximately 100 people. And it came to my skull. You call yourself a healer. Now the lady is dying. You know you can't go to any books because there aren't any books that have within its pages the answer to lockjaw. So you better go into yourself. And what did I come up with? I came up with the answer from within me. The answer was to go to her skull. And I went to her skull. I went to her skull because her jaw

was locked, meaning that the organ that is responsible for her jaw being locked is her brain. I cannot go through her mouth like I usually do to give someone a substance. The mouth is locked. So I have to go where? The nearest point to her brain—her skull. Because her skull is porous. The same herb that I would have given her in her mouth, I put it on her skull wet, hot. And she opened her mouth in 15 minutes or less. So where do you go and find that information? It comes from us but we are not trusting in ourselves, and the reason why we do not trust ourselves is because we don't even trust God. When we stop trusting God, we stop trusting self. Because look, correct me if I'm wrong. Every book on the planet, whether the Bagavad Gita, the Talmud, the Torah or the Koran and not to mention the Holy Bible, it is stated that the herbs are for the healing of the nation. But the followers of these religions when they get sick, where do they go? To the herbs or to a chemical?"

Who can refuse a quick fix when it's available, I thought. Then it hit me. The quick fix is only that, because the symptoms return without fail if the source of the sickness remains. In spite of this revelation, I felt all week—I still do—consciousness plays a role in good health as much as diet. Healing has to start with a decision. Dr. Sebi and I debated that point. He contended a toxic body hampers clear thinking.

"The hypothalamus gland has been interfered with. It cannot process anymore. It cannot decipher. It cannot help you. It has turned against you. But as soon as we abstain from the things that interfere with the hypothalamus gland, there's clarity. Like in the case of the lady dying and I went to her skull, who helped me to go there? I did because my brain was clear enough. And if all of us were to go there you wouldn't need Sebi. We would all be see-

ing. But right now I'm a one-eyed man where everybody is blind. Well, a one-eyed man is king where everybody is blind. But I only have one eye open. This is serious."

I understood. It's a grave situation (no pun intended here, but think about it, how many of our loved ones died of diseases related to improper diet and insufficient information?). In my mind I continued to defend education. You learn to dot your i and cross your t and depend on farmers and health care practitioners to offer appropriate service. Then it dawned on me. Just as Dr. Sebi observed, we're all in the dark.

"As we look at the full picture now, we see that all of the conversations and all of the dialogue and the meetings were based solely on that confused hypothalamus gland. That's why the result is not seeing."

Scientists tell us that if we can reduce the eating of meat by 50 percent it will be enough to change the situation of our planet.

–Thich Nhat Hanh

CHAPTER 5

THE HEALER MAKES A CASE FOR THE NATURAL

Sunday, November 6, 2005, day one in Spanish-speaking Central America. Mayan antiquities in Yucatan, step pyramids in Guatemala. Dole banana plants, rows of them hung wide and long in hues of green and yellow, waiting for processing like Olympians holding before the Parade of Nations. Dr. Sebi, a toastmaster for all things natural, schooled me as we rode past the crops days later, telling me those lush bunches are actually distant cousins to the more nutritious finger-sized original. A finger-sized banana? Never in my life had I eaten one shorter than six inches. My confession didn't surprise Dr. Sebi. More than a few people have disputed his claims about food since the beginning of his career as an herbalist.

As if hearing the doubts all over again he said, and not agitated at all, *"There again, information. If you are in the position or the right place to receive that information and then to process that information properly, to process a piece of information requires what? It requires a level of understanding. But like I said to you earlier, that when a child is at inception, the first thing that takes place is that they remove the child from his original thinking to that of a school. Once entering the school, yes, he would learn the mechanical way of life. But he would disconnect from the cosmic way of life. And what is the need for the cosmic way of life? It is needed because we are a product of this thing called life procession—the Earth. We are a product of such. But when we talk about things like wheat and carrots and beets and turnips, the individual that is able to evaluate that information is an individual who would have had a connection with things outside of the box. In the box, wheat is natural. Outside the box, wheat is unnatural. Why? Because it contains starch. Everything that was made by man has to contain starch as a binder. But starch is carbonic acid."*

❧❧❧

Now I understand his retreat to Honduras. Whistle-blowing the hazards of foodless foods, hybrids, is a one-man show with niche followers and others begging to differ. He told me about the time he answered questions on a radio talk show in New York City. Phone calls flooded the switchboard when he told listeners the carrot, the vegetable claimed to give good eyesight, is unnatural. And just as the news shocked the host and his listeners, it shocked me. I put carrots in my salads. I love carrot cake. I love glazed carrots.

No asthma attack ever followed after eating them. Now I'm hearing for the first time it's a laboratory invention. Here's Dr. Sebi's take on how plant geneticists create hybrids.

"He takes like in a vegetable, the wild yam and the Queen Anne lace, and cross-pollinates them. He opens a sliver of the plant, which is in the stem, and in there he places some of the pollen of another plant, which is the Queen Anne lace and the end product is a carrot. Generally, plants would only pollinate with one of its own kind. And for you to make a third product that was not made by nature, you have to force this other plant to produce a product that it was not designed to do."

"Is the carrot a starch?"

"A carrot has nothing but starch. If you grate carrot and you grind it and you just grind the juice and let it sit, and look what happened at the bottom of the carrot, nothing but starch. It's thick."

Hours would pass before talks of hybrids returned. The press for clarity rewarded me with this information from Dr. Sebi: starch-based foods affect the body's cells and immune system over time. If it's that simple, how did it slip pass us? Dr. Sebi is not the first herbalist. Even he acknowledges the work of people like Paavo Airola, the late nutritionist, naturopathic physician and author of several books on natural healing, including *How to Get Well: Handbook of Natural Healing*. Maybe a better question is how did it get pass food producers, this stray away from the natural and wholesome? Anticipating all my reactions, Dr. Sebi raised his consistent point about formal education, forever looking at it as the main roadblock to proper food consumption.

"What occurs is that we have been taken into a world of philosophy, a world that wants to shape everyone around that one thought pattern, when that is not seen at any time in nature. You find different colors of expression that need different food. You find that the blue vervain is a plant that digests potassium phosphate. And she grows right here in the village and she's a pretty plant. If you want your nerves to be treated properly just think about the blue vervain, the root and the flower. But if you want your bones strong, you have to go the sea moss, and it will strengthen your calcium cells."

His experiences and independence—exposed by lectures, radio shows, the Internet and news sound bites—forbid an embrace of school's regimen. He embraces and advocates, instead, basic acts of nature, including breastfeeding.

"School is necessary in a mechanical society but not in a natural world," he said to a group of visitors to Usha Village in September 2008. *"In the natural world, there is something all together different. In a mechanical world, you ought to drink cow milk. 'Don't give your baby your breast because it was made for a man.' A man told me that in Curaçao. I was there in Curaçao at the time. I took my wife to Curaçao when she was nursing. So I sat her down by the corner with the baby and she's nursing the baby, Kimani. The book says feed your child cow milk. Well, what happened to my breast? I don't see elephants giving their babies lion's milk or horse milk. That elephant gives her babies her milk, not human beings'. Human beings give their babies animal milk. Ok, now listen. To make paper, the intellectuals had to cut down some trees, you understand? They're smart. On paper they put drink cow's milk. But cow's milk will kill you, gradually. That's the*

book. I'm not offering you anything that comes out of a book because if I had, that lady sitting over there, her brother wouldn't
have been cured of diabetes. Because the book says there is no cure.
And there isn't any book that says there is a cure. So I have to use
my brain independent to all. And that's what we should practice,
that independence. How could I allow myself to be taken in by a
school of thought or philosophy that doesn't relate to my momma?
How could I do that? How can I relate to anything that is unlike
my momma? My momma, I came out of her. My momma dictates
everything about my life. I came out of her, so as I look at my
momma and as I look at the outside world, I see my momma obeying certain rules of nature, certain laws. Out of that state that I'm
talking about is where the medicine comes. That's where it comes
from, out of that natural state. That state that God or nature provided for us, we don't have that now."

Separation From the Natural

తతత

I listened to the rhythm of Dr. Sebi's voice, the peaks and
valleys of it. A disciplinarian's tone. I watched him rub his
fingers across his face. The index finger drove his points
home with taps on whatever was closest to it, the mattress,
the nightstand, a thigh, thin air. In all this I saw my father
David, the fireside social analyst, the opinionated voice of
reason, matters of his own health excluded.

He was 72 years old when he died of cardiovascular
disease. A last minute bypass failed. He agreed to try it only
after a lifetime of smoking Camel cigarettes and eating
plates of white rice and butter. As far as I know he never

stepped a foot in Group Health Association for a checkup, no matter how much his family encouraged him to do it. No prostate checkups. No colonoscopies. It was his duty to family, it seemed, to have the high-option health plan he paid for.

"I'm alright. I'm alright. You're going to talk somebody into being sick," Daddy would say, brushing us off. "I'll go when I'm ready." Well, his heart had had enough delays and put him in the hospital April 2001. Doctors were surprised it survived so long in such a weak condition. They prescribed medication for Daddy's heart and obstructed arteries and gave him a prognosis of six months to live. He passed on May 1, 2001.

When Dr. Sebi asked my father's age at death, I answered him like an insubordinate child, as if letting my father know how disappointed I was with his negligence. I blamed stubbornness for his death just as much as the heart disease. Dr. Sebi differed. He said stubborn is not the right word for my father or any other man unaware of how disease grows and ravages the body.

"I find that men that are in their 70s and they're impotent, to them all 70-year-olds are impotent," he said. *"And I find that men in their 30s that are impotent think that all men in their 30s are impotent. So you only have yourself as a barometer. But I want to tell the world that the yardstick they are using is one that is mechanical, because if they just look around and see that everybody is eating the same food and doing the same thing, well, if the diseases occur at the same time, they shouldn't be surprised."*

More silent than easily surprised, and cultured in food ways like other southern folk, Daddy accepted and played life's cards the best way he knew how. No complaints or curiosities about food.

"*But have they ever, any one of them,*" Dr. Sebi continued, *stepped out of the box and see what it would be like? Well, I did at age 30. I know what's in and out of the box. Those that remain in the box they do not know those components that are outside of the box. I see that my friends and my brother, I see that my friends in America, they cannot get away from the box. And I don't blame them and I'm not telling them that they should either. I'm telling them there is life outside of the box they don't know about. And it's a beautiful life.*"

I couldn't help thinking it would be great to hear that kind of contentment every time we talked. Beauty. Knowingness. He blossomed like a new rose in early morning dew when he eased back on his pillows and replaced talks of ill health with good. He offered his own health and return to natural food as evidence of healing that could come.

"*There isn't one Black American that could stand up and say I know the food of my fathers. There isn't one Black Honduran or Caribbean or African that knows the food of their fathers. I concluded that it wasn't a thing that you cooked because they didn't have fire. They didn't have stoves because the body just doesn't digest salt and oil and something hot. The elephant doesn't need anything hot. He doesn't roast his food but lives 400 years — in the forest that is — not the zoo. So we must have eaten the same things that were in our environment. Well, I didn't know the leaves but I do know this — that the plants that are natural, their roots contain energy and that is exactly what I use to reverse disease.*"

Starch is processed to produce many of the sugars in processed food. When dissolved in warm water, starch can be used as a thickening, stiffening or gluing agent, resulting in wheat paste. . . . Wheat starch paste was used by Egyptians to stiffen cloth, weave linen and possibly to glue papyrus. Romans used it in cosmetic creams and hair powder.

–Pliny the Elder

The starch industry extracts and refines starches from seeds, roots and tubers by wet grinding, washing, sieving and drying. The main commercial refined starches are cornstarch, tapioca (cassava), wheat, rice and potato starch.

–Anne Charlotte Eliasson

CHAPTER 6

STARCH, A 400-YEAR CONSUMPTION

I intended to eat natural every day in Honduras but by Saturday, November 12, I'd eaten a fish dinner five nights in restaurants in and on the outskirts of La Ceiba, including a mom and pop eatery in a Garifuna community. Garifunas are descendants of Africans brought to Honduras from the West Indies and Africa in the 17th and 18th centuries. It incensed Dr. Sebi that these offspring were still eating starch-based foods their ancestors assimilated in slavery, cassava a main staple at each meal. Nigerians grate cassava and fry it. They call it gari. Garifunas prepare it in a similar fashion.

Cassava is a starchy tuberous root, rough and light brown much like a potato. In fact, when you peel the rind from cassava it looks like a peeled potato. But in this raw form, cassava—a domesticated plant taken to Africa by Portuguese slave traders—is not only full of starch, but full of cyanide in the form of cyanogenic glucosides called linamarin and lotaustralin.

Uncooked cassava, including its bitter root, can paralyze. Many cassava eaters in West Africa suffer from the paralytic disorder "konzo." Others are afflicted with hypothyroidism and the nerve-damaging disorder, ataxic neuropathy. Iodine deficiency is another problem.

Dr. Sebi showed me "the poison" on my plate. They were fried flat patties with a bland taste, like hard saltless potato chips. Harmless I thought, as I chewed a small corner of one just to experience what riled Dr. Sebi about African diets. I couldn't imagine such a tasteless food effecting Africa's health.

"It's cumulative," he said. *"Eaten over time that's exactly what acid food will do to the human body."*

> *There are today in the subregion several food-crops which many would be willing to bet are indigenous West African foods, but which are in truth exotic, that is, brought in from outside West Africa.*
>
> *–Ifeyironwa Francesca Smith*

He didn't preach while we sat at the table but he was quite blunt and continued.

"The little that I was able to get out of my mother and my father, it has had me at 72 years of age with a healthy body. Sure I feel good. But I can't transpose that to Africans. They're going to die of starvation instead of listening to me. It happened in Zimbabwe. It happened in South Africa. It happened with many places in Africa, including Nigeria. They're eating stimulants. They are

not nourishing their body. This is why impotence is at a very early age in Africa. In Nigeria the average is 30, in Guinea 19."

Starch: It Gels, Swells, It Glues—Think Hardening of the Arteries

၈ၜ၈ၜ၈ၜ

Few fast food restaurants existed when that picture was taken of my godmother Frances. By the late 1960s it wasn't hard to find one on practically every corner in urban America; McDonald's, a favorite stop on my Sunday afternoon car rides with Frances and Leroy. I'd finish one Big Mac, then Frances would buy me another one to take home. Needless to say I was a tad plump in those adolescent days.

Back then obesity and binge eating hadn't become the hot news items they are today. The world is a different place. When he witnessed it in New Orleans in 2005, weight problems didn't surprise Dr. Sebi. Yet he didn't judge the size or health of people he once called neighbors.

"What I saw when I went back to New Orleans was fat people. Fat people, that was before Katrina. In the 50s, New Orleans didn't have fat people. You didn't see fat people in New Orleans. Everybody was slim but they had less fast food and they were less dependent on it and there was a higher degree of sanity among us."

He eased back on his pillows. With fondness and appreciation in his voice, he recounted memories of a simpler, unified time.

"Because I remember going out with fellows and there were no gangs in New Orleans, you know. They were a bunch of

75

fellows and we used to go out and drink our beer once in a while and when we became Muslim we stopped that. But we used to go uptown and buy our gingerbread and goat cheese. Yeah, that was our big meal and we were happy. We were and we were limited see. That's why I owe Islam a lot. But now I find that things I have learned after I left the Nation, I can't return to share with them. It's difficult."

He sighed as his daydream dissolved. Bowtie and suit removed, resignation set in again. He saved some who were obese and diabetic. Others rejected his offerings. Unaffected and in a matter of fact way, he recalled a time of great skepticism after he used his products to cure a Muslim woman of diabetes.

"A sister was treated in San Diego, California. They were about to remove both of her feet. And we gave her the compounds and she recovered. But we told her not to eat the bean pie because the bean pie was too high in glucose and it affected her. She had diabetes. Her feet were black. She has a picture of it. Her name is Sister Paula. She was told by us to discontinue eating lamb or beef or chicken because her blood was septic. To remove the condition and save her, we recommended that she had to stop eating those things. Everything she was told to eat, whether by the Nation of Islam or any other philosophy or religious group, do not eat those things. When she stopped, they called it a miracle. They called it a miracle. The woman has both of her feet. They didn't have to remove them, amputate her feet, and she does not have diabetes."

As it turns out, the navy bean, the legume used in the Nation of Islam's popular navy bean pie, has a high concentration of starch and uric acid, each creating a host of health complications. When uric acid crystallizes it forms gout and kidney stones. The starch residue navy beans leave in the body breaks down the mucous membrane, a protective lining that sweeps toxins out of the body. Chickpeas on the other hand, natural, flavorful, and high in calcium and iron, stand as the best alternative ingredient for bean pie recipes.

Continuing with Sister Paula's story Dr. Sebi recalled, *"She said that she called some of the officials in the Nation and told them about what I did for her and I think that they stopped her right quick. I don't know what was said. But whatever was said was good because like I said, everything is in Divine Order."*

And with that he has retreated to Honduras, accepting the rejection and his track record as it stands, a few thousand cured and satisfied patients. I envisioned mass appeal. I knew his natural products worked, his Eva Salve a mainstay in my bathroom cabinet. I needed to know how they worked in order to inform others. I asked him how he would treat an asthmatic who consistently eats meat, gravy, rice, starch.

"The first thing I would do is what I do for everyone else. To fully understand what we are doing here at the Usha Research Institute, we have to understand, again, life's arrangement. Understanding life's arrangement makes it easier and facilitates reversing a disease. We do not treat the disease like the physician or like the nutritionist. We treat the disease biochemically. We know that when disease is present there's a chemical imbalance. Whether there is diabetes, leukemia or sickle cell, cancer, asthma, whatever the disease, we make the same compounds. But we have to understand what it is we are going to remove from the body to make the individual recover as quick as possible. In the case of an asthmatic person, the bronchial tubes are clogged. His nasal passage suffers

with what? Pneumonia. Quite often he suffers with bronchitis because the body has reached a level of mucous accumulation that is insupportable. I should know. I was born with asthma. I was born with asthma and I had asthma until I was 30. But what I learned about asthmatic people, they are neurotic. The one thing he has lack of is oxygen. Being deprived of oxygen, he fights to stay alive and then any little thing triggers a reaction that is negative. He cannot have that because the oxygen that keeps one healthy and also stable or tranquil, he's being deprived of it. So an asthmatic person, I'm surprised you asked me about an asthmatic person or the disease of asthma because when you describe an asthmatic person's condition, you describe all others because all diseases stem from the accumulation of mucous, whether it's in the bronchial tubes that give you asthma or on the brain that makes you insane. In the prostate gland, prostate cancer. And if the same mucous goes to the pancreas, it's diabetes. So yes, we were able to reduce disease to its least common denominator."

Why it escaped so many of us rolled around in my mind, that simple equation of starch and acid lead to mucous, mucous leads to health problems. Had disease become a family member embraced and accepted? I decided we don't know what Dr. Sebi knows. And even if some of us are aware of the cause of disease, our taste buds are prepped for those stimulants he talks about—comfort foods. I confessed I cheated before traveling to Honduras. I ate broiled barbecue chicken and enjoyed every piece of it. He understood. He said he was a meat eater who had to wean himself off of his cherished lamb chops and eggs benedict. He stressed diet change is crucial on the road to healing.

"That's most necessary and drinking the compounds. The compounds are phosphates. They are carbonates. They are iodides

and they are bromides. What do I mean? They fall into the categories of food and vitalizers. And I'm quoting Shook, Edward Shook. He breaks down the minerals better than anyone I ever read or heard of. But where I differ with Shook is that many times Shook used inorganics to accomplish his goals and he used certain herbs that are unnatural, such as he recommends garlic. And garlic is very acidic. And maybe when he recommended garlic he was recommending for his own gene group. Who knows?"

Dr. Shook is a renowned herbalist and the author of *Advanced Treatise in Herbology*. Rare accolades resonated when Dr. Sebi voiced Edward Shook's name. He spoke as if he celebrated an admired colleague or friend. It was clear Dr. Shook and other herbalists such as Paavo Airola occupied a trustworthy position in his pool of information.

"Paavo Airola, when he wrote his book, How To Get Well, he said that if your ancestors are European, your body is programmed to digest milk. But if you are of African descent or Native American, your body is not programmed to digest milk or lactose. Well, I knew that. I knew that was true. The gorilla cannot eat the polar bear food. He gets sick too. He'll begin to exhibit mucous throughout his body."

I went to a doctor in London and he explained
to me that I had to totally detox the body to get rid
of this pneumonia, bronchial problem. . . . And once
I did all of that my palate actually changed.
So I eat a bit cleaner.

–Tina Turner

CHAPTER 7

FOOD AND THE AFRICAN GENE

Each morning I stepped into Dr. Sebi's hut, I observed a place of great comfort: his body cushioned by pillows on his king-sized bed, his nightstand covered with his herbal products and a half gallon bottle of Fiji spring water. I sat on the futon and watched the news with him if it was on and listened to his bedside analysis of the headlines, usually political headlines. Soccer games diverted his attention more than once. He transformed from Dr. Sebi the healer to Sebi the sports commentator, hurling statistics and player history like thunderbolts. I watched soccer lift him from his pillows and fire him up as much as his herbs. Argentina, Brazil, the UK, he shouted every team's name and praised his favorite players.

When he switched the sports channel to a music channel and let the sounds of jazz ballads play low under our voices, I learned jazz is his other passion. Dr. Sebi is one cool dude talking about and listening to jazz music. I asked him how he could transfer all that enthusiasm to larger groups of people when it comes to healing.

Eager to switch gears to tell me, he said, "*We need to reexamine or revisit the position of our mothers and our fathers. The Bible says honor thy mother and thy father that thy days may be long upon the land. Well that statement doesn't hold true for a gorilla or an elephant. That statement is totally unnecessary because they follow their mother and their father from the day that they are born, the day that she delivered them. That elephant watches what mother eats and so does the gorilla. Now, with the Homo sapiens, the Black race especially, I'm talking for the Black race, the one that they call the African, my gene, we were disconnected from our mothers and our fathers. We don't even know the food that they ate in the jungles of Africa, as they call our place, our dwellings, the jungle. So when the FDA [Food and Drug Administration] wanted to prevent me from distributing my products, I politely asked the FDA, well, maybe the FDA knows the food that is consistent with my cellular predisposition. When you removed the African from Africa did you bring his food with him? Uh oh, that went by. But what people aren't aware of is that those who deprived us of our food they once in a while find us behaving a little bit other than what they would like. And for ourselves, we deprive ourselves of those things that would place us in a comfortable place. But being disconnected without knowing the food of our mothers, so that we could live long upon the land, we eat things that offend our bodies. But even that is in place.*"

"Why is it in place or necessary to eat foods that offend our bodies? How is that going to help African descendants live long upon the land?" I asked him, somewhat surprised by the statement, but certain he would clarify it.

"You know, like Job. He had to get sick before he turned to God. You see, everything is in Divine Order. So the European that brought us here was in Divine Order too. But what he didn't know is that he brought us here to do a job. He didn't even know the job we were going to do. Our job is to heal them. That's right. Just like in the human body, the cells of the brain are made up of copper and carbon. They do not resemble the cells that make up the bones. They are calcium, not to mention the cells that make up the blood. They are iron. They are different cells and they do different things. So the Black race, the Chinese race, the White race, the Eskimo, the Native American, we all were placed here to perform certain duties. But since there was an interruption in our duties that we were supposed to perform, things seem to get out of hand. As we notice carefully, there's unrest all over. So it is necessary for healing. So the healing is coming from us."

He glowed. His eyes beamed as he talked up the preeminent job the Black race was destined to perform. Haughty, unapologetic, and happy to be included in the service, he announced the distinct honor bequeathed to Black people.

"Yes, we are proud to be the servant of the world, the Black race. The angry ones turned out to be the cornerstone that the builders needed to complete the structure. And that's true."

I smiled like a proud parent at Dr. Sebi's proclamation, one of those rare moments he forgave and promoted the collective worth of Black people, returning them to the pedestal, the greatness he often said they should place themselves. Happy for him and for all leaders who resisted him, I knew healing stood at the threshold.

かかか

He had crossed over to good health, leaving other African descendants his age and younger, victims of illnesses he escaped over 40 years ago. I wanted to leave Usha Village armed with an understanding of Dr. Sebi's evolution, thinking that if I laid the first stone a gap could be bridged between him, his skeptics and the impatient. I risked sounding repetitive and asked him to explain the force that drives him.

"I said to you one day curing AIDS and lupus and herpes, blindness and diabetes, that is as easy as ABC for me. You want me to tell you what prepared me to do this. How would I ever know that when I'm in obedience with that energy? I don't know what it is. I'm in obedience to whatever that is. And I don't question it. I never question me. I remember in my dreams I dream that I fly every day. At night I fly. And when I come back on the ground, boy what a relief it is, when I fly. And my life reflects that flying. Because I see things from the top and it becomes easy. Many people are in the forest. They cannot see. I see things from the top. It becomes easy. But when I talk about from the top that becomes confusing now to everyone. By the top I mean that I see things from the top where I can grasp the whole spectrum. I have a larger platform. And I always did that. Like for instance the African people, the African people lived for millions of years without the aid of money. Now the African people find themselves needing money to feed themselves. The African needs to starve to death. That in itself is telling them that they have departed so far from

their ancestors that now they need money, something that was never part of the repertoire of Africa—money. You can't even eat if you don't have money."

He sat up on the edge of his bed lambasting and chastising, driving his points home with the proverbial thrust of his index finger. Underneath the outcries though, I heard urgent pleas to reverse the fatalities, reverse them with proven solutions.

"We came from a people that didn't have any money. We could live life without money. We could design societies. All it takes is some mud and some grass and we could build empires again. Because we did it right here in Usha Village. All these huts are mud. They're mud and grass. And we could do it again as easy as that."

Bold, brave methods are necessary to turn things around I thought, even though the food industry around the world is a multibillion dollar entity. But when I researched African and African American health news and reports, I learned an expedient lesson from the World Health Organization and the United Nations: people in developing countries eat whatever the socioeconomic climate allows them to eat—more often than not inexpensive and quick-distribution bulk foods, starch-rich bulk foods, including the highly toxic cassava.

"With me, it would not be that if I was the president of an African country," Dr. Sebi suggested when we talked about how to move food consumers and producers into the knowledge of life-sustaining foods, no matter what the costs.

"I would show them but with my understanding of this point now. I'm not saying that the presidents of Africa know what

I know. They were interested in civics and politics. Mine was a different giving. It was healing. But as an individual citizen of a country, America or Africa or Honduras —I am indebted to America just as much as Africa or Honduras —I would make certain suggestions. So now we're going to change this format. The paradigm has shifted right? The method has to change. Am I right? So now that Africa finds itself at a deficit financially, well, just go back to the ways of our fathers. Let's go back to the forest and find the herbs that have the energy. We can begin to experiment with new organically electric food."

༄༄༄

Even with all Dr. Sebi knows about African slavery: the separation of Africans from original food groups and all the diseases that sprang up due to that separation, disgust never set in. He spoke with a prophet's stance, with an eye on the future.

"I'm not saying Black America is handicapped because it was willfully done. We were placed in a condition that had to happen. Now where are you going to take off from here? Well, I don't know. But what happened to Black America or an African in America is that they were removed. And after that removing from Africa, what' going to happen after that, well I know it is out of the hands of those that brought us and those who participated. But one thing is certain there is a new message on the horizon —the healing of the nation. From the healing of the nation we know that we are now on the right track because it brings peace. It brings health. And that is what we had when we were taken away from Africa. We didn't wear glasses. And there were no fat people. All

of the sketches and all of the pictures shown about Black slaves you never saw fat ones."

He didn't mock obese people. I sensed his concern. But surrounding the concern was opposition from others and I gathered that agitated him when he talked about it. I saw his point. Since he embodies all he advocates, there shouldn't be opposition but acceptance.

Unlicensed, self-taught, confident and secure in his prognosis, Dr. Sebi surveyed the landscape of meat and starch eaters as if an x-ray of malignancies hung in front of him.

"Well, the food that we eat is the very substance that causes the whole hormonal structure of the body to go haywire because it's of an acid base. So you're going to get acid thoughts. I listened to the guru. Well, I was not encouraged to any great extent because I know that words do not put you in a cosmic balance. It is the food that you eat that would reconnect you with energies of life and then words are unnecessary because you could see. You're connected. Like the eagle. How come the eagle could make that nest? How could the beaver make the dam? The spider makes his web? Because it is coded. But you have to be cleansed of the poisons that you were unaware were entering your brain. So now we have to perform, what do you call it, a catharsis? How do you do that? How do you

Tot (funio fufu) on the other hand being a cereal product is a more nutritious fufu compared to cassava and yam products like eba, amala or pounded yam and so constitutes a nutritious addition to the food list for fufu eating groups.

—Ifeyironwa Francesca Smith

89

tell someone in Mississippi or even in Honduras or even in Africa, around Nigeria, 'Say Nigerians, you can't eat gari.' Man, he's going to beat you in your head. You can't tell him that. So, he has chosen death over life. That is what glucose will do to the hypothalamus."

"But we don't know," I said, defending our ignorance.

"Well that makes it better. You don't know."

"Why does that make it better?"

"Because you're enjoying your poison. You see, if you knew that you were eating it, you'd be chastising yourself every day, because you're unaware. But if you don't know, you're enjoying it. 'Yeah man, I like this chop. Man, I'm diggin' this.' I remember when I liked my pork chop. I remember when I loved my pork chops. And I remember when I liked eggs, eggs benedict. So when I came into the understanding that these things are dangerous to the body and I would go back to eat them once in a while, I was punished because I know I was doing the wrong thing like before."

"How were you punished?"

"I felt bad."

"Oh, your body reacted."

"I felt bad because I felt like I'm jive. I'm weak."

"For eating the poisons again?"

"That I know are poisons."

࿔࿔࿔

"The Black man was never supposed to eat meat," He professed. *"The Black race cannot assimilate meat nor alcohol.*

Why? Because over the 31 years of my research, when my genetic group that I represent, the so-called Black man, the African, I find that when they come with diabetes, lupus, herpes, and this is all manifested in one body, in less than a fortnight, all of the diseases disappear. But we have to abstain from eating the very substance that made our body sick, which is the blood of the animal. Meat was never supposed to be consumed by the Black race. But maybe other races, like I was told in Atlanta. I was told in Atlanta by a Native American at the lecture that I gave recently in the month of October, this Native American said, 'Dr. Sebi did you know that they found a very rare enzyme in the blood of the buffalo and that enzyme prevents the individual from getting cancer and this is why the Native American people have a very low rate of cancer incidence?' So there is a rare enzyme in the blood of the buffalo. I said that may be true for Native Americans, but I represent a different gene group and in that difference a lot will be seen and could happen. What occurs is that the difference has never been treated. Over the last 500 years, the intent is to group all of us in obedience to a philosophy. But that does not hold true for the plants, and the flowers and the planet. Even the birds, they all obey the dictate that was designed to support their life and their cellular group. Like it is mentioned, the gorilla does not eat meat. Where did the gorilla get that message from? He didn't go to school to learn from a nutritionist that his cells are not made to digest meat. It is encoded in the gorilla, like everything else. But when we talk about encoded, what is it that we are talking about? We are talking about an expression or an electrical connection with life. That electrical connection gives you the ability to make a decision that is equitable and good. But when we disconnect from that electrical connection we make mistakes. We are vulnerable. Because it is seen that the Homo sapien puts meat and cheese in his mouth. I'm referring to those who represent the gene of Africa. But by the time they get to 45 the doctor politely tells them, 'Well, I find that you are suffering with hypertension. Your pressure is a little high and by the way, did you know that your PSA is a little high?' The Black man is totally unaware that he's obeying a dictate that had nothing to do with the history of his cellular predisposition."

God's Wheat, Spelt

ৡৡৡ

Dr. Sebi introduced me to spelt bread when I stopped by his suite in Los Angeles. It looks like a light brown multigrain bread and has a nutty taste. The taste pleased me so much that now, with the exception of an occasional croissant, spelt bread is the only bread I eat, usually as toast or in a grilled cheese sandwich—almond cheese.

Speaking about today's fast processed, mass marketed brands, Dr. Sebi trumpeted, *"God made spelt. God didn't make wheat or white bread."* Why does he claim spelt the best grain, spelt bread the best bread, where you'll

A study at the diabetes clinic of Grady Memorial Hospital in Atlanta, Georgia, found that the primary reason for patients not following food recommendations was that the recommended diet was not familiar to them and contained unfamiliar food choices.

–Karmeen D. Kulkarni

find in some brands tiny spelt kernels baked in the bread? Spelt is difficult to process and cultivate like fast-bred, high volume modern wheat. That's good because what's retained in spelt harvesting—nutrients, high fiber, B complex vitamins—complements and nourishes the immune system. And here's an interesting spelt fact I learned that aligns itself with Dr. Sebi's affinity for natural foods: spelt dates back to 5,000 BC and its tough husk, even today, protects it from pollutants and insects so well, that spelt growers rarely use pesticides on the crop.

That reacquaintance with Dr. Sebi in 2005 opened up a wellspring of information about food and hybrids he's talked about in over 20 years of speeches. When I accepted his invitation to visit Usha Village, I decided the trip would serve a dual purpose: help Dr. Sebi with his autobiography and gather as much information as possible about available natural, unhybridized foods. I wanted to be clear about alkaline foods and acid foods. I planned to go to Honduras and absorb his knowledge, retrieve life-saving gems he claimed all of us owned a long time ago.

He was more than happy to divulge all he knew when my crusade arrived at Usha Village.

"What are some good alkaline foods?" I asked him on the first day of recording our conversations.

"Mushrooms. Then you have spelt. You have quinoa. Those are the grains. Quinoa, tef. The other one from the desert of Mali, which is fonio. And then you have the amaranth. These are the natural grains, alkaline."

"What other foods? These are grains. What vegetables?"

"Natural spinach that we have growing here at the Village, that you could also have in the United States. I have a natural spinach that runs on a vine that produces a flower."

I wanted to know how collard greens rated with Dr. Sebi. I'm the offspring of South Carolina-born parents and collards were a staple vegetable in our home. "What about collard greens?"

"No."

"What?"

"That's very hard on your digestive system."

"Collard greens?"

"Most definitely."

He didn't flinch. I assumed the time needed to cook the leaves influenced his answer. In fact, the cooking time for collard greens is longer than other leafy high fiber vegetable due to the toughness of the leaves. And the 20- to 30-minute cooking time causes the water to absorb most of the nutrients. When my mother saved leftover collards, she'd save some of the water, better known to southern folks as pot liquor.

I relented and moved on, sensing it best not to belabor a point with the good Dr. Sebi. "Kale? Mustard greens?"

"Mustard greens are more digestible. So is kale. Turnip greens too but not collards. They are very hard, very hard."

"Spinach."

"Spinach has a lot of oxalate acid."

"That's not good?"

"Well, it's questionable."

His answers seemed more eccentric by the minute and I dare not speak for Dr. Sebi, but oxalate acid has pros and cons. Oxalates occur naturally in not only plants, including collards and spinach, but in human beings. But kidney stones found in humans contain calcium oxalate, crystallized calcium, and that fact may influence Dr. Sebi's reluctance to support our beloved spinach.

I probed. The goal was to understand the difference between acid and alkaline food. Why did it matter?

"The starchy foods of course are peanuts and what else?"

"They have carbonic acid. But we shouldn't even single out one or two of the items that you mentioned. Anything that has an acid base will undermine your immune system immediately, primarily because it's an acid base. It's going to eat you up. It's going to weaken the system. It's going to weaken the red blood cells. Acid causes the central nervous system to contract, which again causes you to go into a state of despair. So what are the acids? Well, you just walk into a supermarket and walk out with a coconut. Everything you left behind is acid. But there are health food stores that have mushrooms, the Portobello. You also have the oyster mushrooms. You also have spelt bread. You could select, in the vegetable kingdom, all the greens, except the collard greens. See, I make it easy. But now you need to be educated as to how you're going to prepare these things. Ah-h, now you call for a whole big institute. I came to heal people of diseases. Now I find myself having to address a whole lot of other things. Well, I'm not qualified for that. That is for the leaders who have placed themselves in the position of leadership. I am not a leader."

Whatever thought or activity is carried on by the individual, if it is in accordance with natural evolution, if it is in accordance with the cosmic purpose, it creates an influence that is in accordance with the natural laws.

–Maharishi Mahesh Yogi

Chapter 8

Alfredo Bowman is Dr. Sebi the Healer

"I don't consider myself strong or weak. I don't know what strong is or weak. I never lived that. These are some of the things that most people don't know about Sebi. Sebi is not, was never poor and he will never be rich. Sebi, he doesn't know what strength is, no. He doesn't know what weakness is. He just lives. I just live. I know I'm an individual that most people like, and I'm an individual where there are some individuals that don't like me and both are right. They interpret me, they perceive me differently. So, about strength, I'm afraid of that word because I consider myself a pussycat."

He was at times and I cherished those moments, privy to the unusual joy and contentment of a Black man in love with his herbs. He caressed his plants, adored them as much as a lioness fancies her cubs.

"It's a pretty plant. It grows right here in the village," he said when he introduced me to the blue vervain. As far as I

could tell only his grandmother Mama Hay occupied the same pedestal as this honored plant. I suppose I should thank her for the privilege to see Dr. Sebi raw, to see him childlike and free in his love of plants. And I'm not alone. Others have witnessed his passion. A biochemist sat in the audience at one of his lectures and questioned him about how he uses herbs in his products.

"The man asked me, 'Do you intend to isolate the active ingredients of the plants and apply them to your therapeuticals?' Where do you think this biochemist got his information? From his books, right? From his schools, right? I know that. The active ingredient. There are 102 minerals in everything that exists that is natural. If you take clouds and take them to a laboratory and break them down, you'll find 102 minerals. If you take the soil and you analyze it, 102 minerals. Sea salt, 102. The human body, 102. Well, anything that is unnatural doesn't have that arrangement, like carrots and beets and rice and beans. They don't have that. This man is asking do you intend to isolate the active ingredient. Let us assume that this circle is the burdock plant. Burdock has 102 minerals. But in the arrangement of 102, there is one that is called the active ingredient. That is the one that is more in percentage. There is calcium. There is phosphorous. There is iron. There is magnesium and zinc. But they all are distributed proportionately. But iron is the largest one. Out of all the minerals, iron occupies the majority of the structure. What he's asking me is do I intend to remove the iron over here by itself and leave the 101 behind. But in the arrangement how much are there? 102. But if I remove 1, I leave 101 behind, right? But this one was in an arrangement with the other 101 to supply it with what it needs to exist. If you remove it, sir, it becomes a protoplasmic poison. The man looked at me and realized that the school didn't teach him *that. The school came out of philosophy, not out of seeing. When you see and when you believe—two different things. When someone educates us is one thing but when you see, it's all together different. So when the man said do you intend to isolate the active ingredient I said no sir, absolutely not. Life doesn't express itself in one. You've got to use the whole plant, not part of it. And the man said thank you Dr. Sebi."*

Leadership

৯৵৯৵৯৵

By Thursday, November 10, I learned leaders step straight out of a mother's womb in Honduras. I was riding with Dr. Sebi in his truck one morning and I watched little boys and little girls, literally little boys and girls no older than 3 or 4 years old, walk alone beside the paved two-lane road near Usha Village. Some carried a bag or two of items from wood-slatted roadside stores. Other toddlers walked yards behind what could have been a faster walking mother or father holding a sibling. They walked with a purpose, look-ing neither left nor right, these baby adults, unfazed by traf-fic or mules on the road. I moaned and winced at the sight. A 3-year-old alone on the road? I felt an urge to scoop them up to safety, every single child. Dr. Sebi quickly reminded me that that child was him, same age, 70 years ago. Without regret and without fail, he said his childhood independence shaped his success as a healer as much as it shaped his feel-ings about leadership.

"Yes, of course. I was happy to know that the perspective that I was using was affording me the privilege to reach that level of offering. I was happy because in the past I had visited Dr. Woo, a Chinese. He didn't heal me. I went to some Black herbalists in California. They didn't heal me. And then I went to the chiropractor and he didn't heal me. So naturally when I put the compounds together, I trusted my judgment. Why? Because I selected plants whose molecular structure is complete, which deems them electrical; and so is the human body. But when the individual that had AIDS was cured, then I was encouraged to know, or when the blind man was seeing I was further encouraged. So you see I had to be excited. But the excitement is giving way to reality."

"And that reality is?" I asked.

"That what I wanted is one thing and what is forthcoming from my brothers and sisters is another. It's totally different. I am not talking about those of us who are sick, because the people have come in large quantities, sure. They have been supporting me for the last 30 plus odd years. Sure, and I give all of you thanks, of course. But we are talking about the people who have taken responsibility to lead others. Those were the people. Those are the people that represent the reality that I'm talking about. The reality is yes, Dr. Sebi can cure AIDS and lupus and herpes. But yes, on the other hand, it doesn't mean anything because we're not going to support him. I accept."

"How are you not supported?"

"I don't believe that it's necessary to mention names. I'm talking about every Black American leader. That's who I'm talking about. Because they claim that they are leaders. So naturally one expects for a leader to help the flock out of the disease state to a better state. They, not I, took the position of leadership. So if you're going to lead a people, and from the people came the solu-

tion to one of the major problems that beset the community and you do not act on it, what is the message that you are sending? That is the reality."

ॐॐॐ

Comfort and trust settled in by Friday evening, pushing us well beyond Dr. Sebi's bedtime. He slouched on his pillows and rested horizontal on his bed like a well fed lion on a tree limb, unaffected by our little eavesdropping lime green gecko hovering on the ceiling. It scampered across the walls every night we talked, but by Friday the tropic's lizard and one or two others failed to arouse my curiosity as it had my first and second nights at Usha Village. And like the legs of those geckos that scurried about, Dr. Sebi's energy churned him from one topic to another. The top of the list—social and political leaders skeptical about his healing and unaware of the correlation between food and disease.

"There has never been an educator in America that has done research in neuropathology associating the disease with the food that goes in the person's mouth. That research has never been done. So what rule do they have to challenge? You see nobody could challenge me on this planet because I have accomplished what no one else has accomplished. So where's the room for challenge? Since there is no challenge there is ridicule. But I say this, the glucose on the brain is shown when all of the leaders of America that know about the entities of healing and have turned their backs on it. I can openly say they all know that I exist. I have proof of that too. When I was taken to the Harlem State Building [Adam Clayton Powell State Office Building] to address AIDS, the African American War on AIDS in 1989, I told them that I had the

cure for AIDS and they laughed. I went to Detroit and I told Dr. Whitner I had the cure for sickle cell anemia. He laughed. I went to some of the biggest leaders in America. So now Dr. Sebi knows that healing someone with diseases is one thing but changing their thought pattern, well. So if there's any change, well, hope there'll be. But changes cannot be accomplished and will not be forthcoming if the diet has not changed. And if the diet is not changed I will live long enough to see that in the next 30 years, America is not going to change."

I risked another disturbance. I defended American leaders. Without trepidation I said leaders shouldn't be blamed for the same inexperience most of us harbor when it comes to food and disease. I said food habits are generational, passed down from great grandmothers and grandfathers, caregivers focused on keeping bellies full with available food, natural or laboratory-made. Who, besides scientists, knows an orange carrot is a genetically-engineered product? What father or mother knows they're feeding their family cross-pollinated hybrid foods?

Dr. Sebi listened, like a professor allowing his student to debate a point, he listened. He reflected. I braced myself. I sensed a counterpoint coming.

ॐ ॐ ॐ

He built a two-feet wide canal full of water from his hot spring and let it run down the middle of his 14 cabins, 7 cabins on each side, including one dedicated to its most famous guest, Lisa "Left Eye" Lopes. When I stepped outside my cabin every morning, I sat on the canal's edge and let ripples of water cover my feet. Warm, soothing, with a pH no less than 8.0, Dr. Sebi's water felt more like lotion than water from a hot spring. And that same body of water provided a welcome respite after talks of leadership had erupted into volcanic tirades. He had lived his share of opposition with leaders around the world and decided he needed only one leader—Sebi.

"When I went to Zimbabwe and I showed these people with diagnostic sheets from laboratories that they support, and they rejected it, I knew they were disrespectful. And that is all I needed to see. I'm not going to make any excuses for Africa. No. There's only one country in Africa that I would return to and that's the country of Guinea. No other. Why? Because they blatantly disrespected the entity. I loved it because it tells me about their conscience and their compassion. It tells me about their inner self. Yet, they tell the world that they would do anything to combat the ravages of AIDS. That is far from the truth. There isn't any African country but one that is interested in the eradication of AIDS or any other disease. That's Guinea. No other country is interested in that. How do I know? Because they know about me and they know I cure AIDS."

He was preoccupied with his strained relationship with Zimbabwean leaders, so much so that he never mentioned the troubles he saw in Zimbabwe when he travelled there in 2004: Zimbabwe's dire need of the help he could offer, life expectancy for males and females no higher than 45 years, the AIDS crisis preventing a population growth higher than 0.8%, and major shortages of food and health supplies throughout the country due to drought and economic sanctions imposed on the country by the United States and Europe. Besides that, Africa faced and still faces challenges with its own healers.

When I researched traditional healers in Africa, the words witch doctor and rogue herbal healers came up. Dr. Sebi never talked about this issue, but I assumed the stigma attached to these labels met up with him in Africa and produced some of the ill feelings. It's a delicate situation. Both sides—healers and African public health officials—have valid opinions when it comes to healing the sick. I found a Zimbabwean organization that supports the practice and beliefs of both groups is ZINATHA, the Zimbabwe National Traditional Healers Association. For more than 20 years, ZINATHA has regulated and provided networking assistance to herbalists and indigenous healers (practitioners whose services pre-date modern medicine in Zimbabwe). Maybe that's the thorn between Zimbabwe and Dr. Sebi. Zimbabwe's indigenous healers prevent her full scale acceptance of what Dr. Sebi has to offer.

In Malawi, officials want to ban herbal healers. They favor pharmaceutical antiviral medications and insist AIDS victims take them. South Africa, like Zimbabwe, wants healers regulated, a position that seems to favor Dr. Sebi's work. I suppose for mass healing to take place some level of mediation is required.

৵৵৵

I counted on a high spirited time with Dr. Sebi. I remembered the first lectures. But I didn't expect to be a vicarious player in his memories of Africa. As the hours with him passed, my questions and comments became more guarded. I wanted to prevent another Zimbabwe. Sometimes I succeeded, sometimes I didn't. Like the time I said he would have to put his expertise in writing to be validated by the Black community. A matador couldn't have agitated a bull more. Et tu, Beverly? *An all expense paid trip to Central America and you show gratitude with talks of validation? The gall!* That moment I became one of them—the naysayers, the skeptics, Brutus. He pushed forward from his pillows and hurled innuendos across the room like a quarterback sneak, disguising his attack on an insult, a perceived insult. If I ever needed someone to clarify or back up what I meant, surely that was the time. I used diplomacy to shield me when I said the written word tends to authenticate the spoken word in the minds of some readers. He panned my face, searching for some semblance of loyalty and appreciation. Finding it, he eased back on his pillows wrapped in the understanding I lacked the knowledge of his experiences with indifference, where there should be support.

I breathed a sigh of relief, sensing a tough love going on between Dr. Sebi, leaders and Africa. Throughout my week with him, he put aside conflicts on how to heal the continent, and identified that heritable land as the source of all he accomplished in life.

"In the house that I was raised I always heard that self-preservation was the first law of nature. Being that I am of an African genetical structure, an African heritage, I couldn't very well say Japan or Europe. I had to say Africa. That is the beauty of each and every one of us that represent that gene. That is the beauty. So with me saying I'm going to go to Africa, it was an automatic thing. It wasn't something I had to think about. It was automatic because it was ingrained in the house in which I was raised."

"Your mother's or Mama Hay?" I asked.

"*Mama Hay.*"

"What did she say about Africa?"

"*Well, all she had to say was that we are Africans and she kept saying that. We are Africans. We are not Mayans. We are not Native Americans. We are Africans brought to this part of the world.*"

"She told you that?"

"*Um hum. It's as simple as that. I'm an African. I'm not an African-Honduran, no. I'm an African in Honduras.*"

༺༺༺

He inherited his grandmother's free-speaking soul. He said she often advised him to walk naked if he ever found himself without provisions. Nothing more, simply make do with what's available.

"*That was sufficient,*" he said, resigned that whatever his grandmother taught him it helped him survive.

"*I interpreted it in a way that she wanted me to receive it, you see. But in America that's arrogance because that's how they perceive me, as arrogant, when I talk the way I talk. In fact, it was recently my mother told me when she looked at the tape when I was speaking in Washington, I was very angry at the audience. And she told me that I was the only angry person there. But she understood why I was angry. I was dissatisfied because why should I have a piece of information and no one else in the community has that information? That doesn't put me in a good position. It puts me in a vulnerable position. Because it tells me how weak we are, how vulnerable the whole race really is. Because in*" *the forest what one gorilla knows, all gorillas know. What one Black man in the forest knows, every Black man knew. Not now."*

And it incensed him that others have lost the knowledge of healing. I was learning the source of his agitation with others, all the contentions on his journey with natural healing. They unfolded in front of me and exposed a barrier that stood between him and conventional thinking, even as early as his childhood.

He recounted, *"As I look back in retrospect I could remember this: people would ask my grandmother, 'Miss Ann, what's going to happen to Fred?' My grandmother would say, 'I don't know.' 'Miss Ann, what's going to happen to Fred?' 'I don't know.' 'Fred, what is it you want to be?' they would ask me. I said I don't know, because I don't know. I'm only 8 or 9. I didn't know what I wanted to be. 'But why don't you go to school, Fred?' 'I don't like it.' As simple as that. I didn't like it. Ok. What I see now that avails me the privilege to look at things from outside the box, I was never in the box. Because I had the freedom to think as I wish for myself. And that is something children are not afforded. That's the one thing Mama Hay afforded me, the environment to think for Fred."*

A nonconformist in childhood and adulthood. Debates, questions, analyses of conventional views all his life.

"Everybody resonates differently," he said. *"And everybody comes with a good message afforded in a different way. My grandmother wasn't better than your mother or grandmother either. My grandmother isn't better or worse than any other grandmother. My grandmother just resonated differently. This is what we have failed to see. We always measure things with up and down and good and bad and in between. No. Things are different. How can you compare a lion with a jaguar? There are dif-*

ferent animals, to do different things, to live in different geographies. That's another thing about geographies. Plants live geographies. You would never find a coconut plant growing in Canada. But you'll never find burdock growing in Honduras. So you see, these simple, natural cosmic rules and laws, we don't know about. And those laws are the ones that still continue to govern things. So you see, Mama Hay obeyed the laws of life and she transposed that into her grandson."

Mama Hay encouraged independent thinking. She laid an unshakeable foundation of self-preservation. Yet she and her daughter Viola, Dr. Sebi's mother, fed him the same food southern American mothers fed their families 70 years ago.

"Rice, beans, potatoes, yams, hog feet, hog head, chicken, oxtail. Everything that you see on the table hasn't changed in 500 years. But I was able to get away from it because someone in Mexico said I wasn't honoring my mother or my father. And he stopped me from eating meat and because of that I was able to see the other part of it. But she cooked the same thing. That's all she had. And even if she wanted to cook something else, they didn't have spelt in Honduras."

And that's the key, the availability of proper foods. Once communities in the United States like Appalachia, the Mississippi Delta, African and Latin American countries gain, or shall I say re-gain, knowledge about spelt, kamut, tef, wild rice and sea vegetables, the challenge is how to distribute these foods in a way that not only meets the economic demands of the people, but the demands of Earth and the climate. Cassava is an inexpensive crop that flourishes in drought-prone countries, but cassava harvested in a drought is far more toxic than at any other time of the year.

It was just recently I understood why Dr. Sebi's prescriptions for healing placed him at odds with leaders of developing countries. His stance, nutrition; developing countries', economy and the residue of colonialism.

Nonetheless, as young Alfredo living in rural Honduras, notions of voyages around the world, including Africa, intrigued him.

"So you went to South Africa for the first time in your 20s," I asked, eager to hear about his global excursions.

"*Um hum.*"

"Why South Africa?"

"*I was a merchant seaman. I had to go where the ship goes.*"

"You became a merchant seaman because you could travel to Africa?"

"*Because I could travel the world.*"

"The world?"

"*Um hum.*"

"By being a merchant seaman you would eventually end up going to Africa."

"*Most certainly.*"

"What does a merchant seaman do?"

"*It does a lot of things. The ship takes cargo. You have people work in the steward department. You have people work in the deck department. You have people work in the engine department. I chose the engine.*"

"Why?"

"*Because I was always interested in engines.*"

In a conversation in his hut one morning, Dr. Sebi recounted that his travels as a merchant seaman often took

him to places where he learned of plants he would eventually use as an herbalist.

*"I learn about the use of the elderberry in Yugoslavia.
This man was playing the piano and he was drinking out of his
glass and he was very happy. So I asked the bartender what was
that? And he looked at the bottle—elderberry. He said, 'That man
is not going to get tired because he drinks elderberry.' And many
years later when I was assisting someone in Los Angeles, a lady in
her 85th year, she was very weak, I remembered the elderberry."*

Reflections on the Elderly and the Young at Usha Village

సౌసౌసౌ

By Wednesday, November 9, I'd grown accustom to Dr. Sebi's emotions volleying from cordial to angry, from toler-
ance to solitude. His was an inconsistent bedside manner.
Yet our reunion endured on a personable level.

He decided to introduce me to his 92-year-old
mother Viola. Matun joined us in an afternoon ride to visit
her in La Ceiba. I sat in the backseat of the truck switching
my journalist hat with the one more tourist. Agua Caliente
mountains hovered miles high in shades of green from forest to blue green. Between the road and the foothills, about
every half mile or so, bluish gray smoke rose above piles of
burning bushes and trash. Horses and mules grazed and
yes, the usual lone child or two sauntered along. They were
sights that repeated themselves miles down the stretch of
road. But one particular patch of brush and fauna caught

Dr. Sebi's attention. He slowed the truck down and gently nodded at the spot where hip hop singer Lisa "Left Eye" Lopes crashed and died in a car accident in 2002. A numbing silence filled the truck as we passed the area. Then, in my own quiet and private thoughts, I mourned the loss right there in the truck.

I enjoyed Lisa's music. I listened to it, rocked to it, and like a proud big sister, watched her and her singing group TLC perform in music videos on television. In my mind I started to hear a slow tinny horn crescendo into *Creep*, one of my favorite TLC songs (but not one of Lisa's I'd find out later). I was suddenly transported back to my apartment in Washington, D.C. in 1994. I sat still and let my mind's eye follow TLC's slick hip hop dance moves. Legs swiveled, bodies gyrated, Lisa's handstands and body flips theatrical and in sync with *Creep's* rhythm. Such talent, such wonderful vivacious talent, I thought.

When Dr. Sebi informed me he and Lisa had been friends in the United States and Lisa journeyed to Usha Village to rest, I deemed it divine providence that Lisa and I shared an acquaintance and an interest in herbal healing.

As we passed palm trees and plants rising high and thick against Agua Caliente's mountains, I returned to my moment with Dr. Sebi and segued into a comment that his tropical home base complemented all that he stood for.

His hands clutched the top of the truck's steering wheel.

He said, "*If I am not in compliance and obedience with life I would not exhibit the energy I exhibit now. And I'm not saying I'm batting a thousand either. But the little effort, after coming from a very shaky foundation with asthma, diabetes, impo-*

tence, blindness at an early age with glasses on my eyes, to reach 72 healthy, I must have done something because I was led to understand the arrangement of life. But how many brothers and sisters in America know this?"

He stared down the middle of the road, his eyes fixed on it. In an urgent voice he continued.

"And this is why for us to really get over, get over meaning what, from the state of disease to ease, that jump, that crossing over is called dembali. But I cannot talk to, I could hardly talk to people in my own family. And what about the hip hop group? They are our young brothers and sisters that need to be told that the degree that they are traveling, the speed is going to affect their lives in a very short period of time because they are exhibiting diseases that were never seen before until like 70 or 80, like diabetes. Diabetes? Everybody have diabetes. I don't care what age you are. You have diabetes. You're going to hear it all around. Three, four, five, six born with diabetes. Children are born with diabetes."

Alfredo Bowman—Ward of the State

࿎࿎࿎

He had had his own bouts of weakness, mental weakness. His strength in herbs and natural healing would come later. After listening to all he said about independent thinking and self-preservation, I found it hard to imagine his invincible constitution laid low by mental illness in his merchant seaman days. He reassessed the condition as if it happened yesterday.

"I was considered to be a schizophrenic and paranoid in 1961. This can be researched in New Jersey, in Paramus, New Jersey where I was hospitalized. And I remember being in this place and thinking about my life, how I, Alfredo, not Sebi yet, I was Alfredo. How I, without knowing, neglected my body and find myself in a mental health institution. But even though I was in an institution being treated something in me kept saying you're not going to give in to this. And I wouldn't drink the medication. I would pretend that I was drinking it. And I would throw it away."

"Why did you agree to being admitted?"

"It's not that I agreed. I didn't agree to go in. This happened because I was on my way to India on a ship and for some reason there was some oil on the deck of the ship and I slipped on it and it hurt my spine. And they took me off the ship. But while I was off the ship the doctor at the hospital detected something in me. His medical report, his final analysis was that I was schizophrenic and paranoid."

"On the ship?"

"Absolutely right. This happened in the Azures Islands. The ship put me off in the Azures. The ship was on the way to India but I didn't reach India. I am still looking for those monies due to me now. This is 1961 that that happened. When they shipped me back to the United States I was shipped back handcuffed to a stretcher."

"Why? What were you doing to make them think you were mentally off base?"

"I don't know."

"Were you saying something?"

"I don't remember that. But as you know, that when you are sick mentally or emotionally you are totally unaware as to

115

your behavior. But I was aware sufficient enough to walk out of that hospital. Malcolm was the one who took me out. Malcolm X, the Malcolm that everybody talks about. You see at the time I was a Muslim. So I went to the orderly and I asked him for 10 cents. And he said, 'Who are you going to call your friend, your Martian friends? Oh, Bowman has some Martian friends.' I say yes, I have some Martian friends."

"Where did that come from?"

"Well, he invented that, the orderly. So he gave me the dime and I went to the phone and I called the Mosque. The brother by the name of Captain Yusef Shaw answered the phone. He remembered me vaguely but he did remember something of me when I came from New Orleans to Number 7, Mosque Number 7 in New York. He remembered me. So he said he would tell the Minister. The next day, which was Saturday, I had two bald headed Muslim lawyers there and they took me out. That's right. They even gave me a state test, the sanity test, and I passed it in front of them. But I knew even though I passed the test that something was occurring in me that needed to be treated. I was aware of that."

"Do you think the doctors were picking up on that?"

"Right. Whatever they picked up for them to conclude that I was mentally helpless or ill, was true, that I didn't know about. I didn't know but I felt it. I don't know what I projected. That I will never know. I was very uneasy. I was totally dissatisfied and I used to cry every evening."

Many times I wanted to express shock at what this articulate world traveler and nutritionist told me. I held it back thinking it would offend him, and because he sat before me grounded in good mental and physical health, though his emotional pendulum that week swung from incendiary to the comedic. Maybe that was the hint of his past.

As I think back on that part of our conversation, it felt more like a psychological profile than a biographical interview.

"Your lifestyle?" I asked. "Maybe it's because you weren't doing what you were supposed to do."

"If I wasn't supposed to be crying and going through those trials and tribulations I was going through, how was those things occurring?"

"Why do you think they were occurring?"

"Because they were supposed to occur."

"They were supposed to?"

"If they weren't supposed to occur they would not have been occurring. Now, the interpretation of the occurrence, that's a different thing. I never give occurrences interpretations. I just know that whatever occurs in my life was supposed to occur and those occurrences brought me to this end."

"To where you are today."

"To where I am today."

తతతత

I kept the recorder rolling even though by Friday, November 11 the conversations turned somewhat repetitive. In his hut or on the road in his truck, I kept it rolling. I thought he might suggest other little known food and healing options. I didn't want to miss a revelation about his past or plans for his future. The recorder didn't get a chance to record much of the latter.

"I don't plan anything. How can I plan my life? When I was born, I grew up without education. If anybody on this planet that couldn't bargain for anything on any level of endeavor should

be me. Because I didn't have any of the tools that are required by society to reach a certain level of expression. I don't have any of those tools. I was never graded by anyone to see whether I failed, except when I went to get the test for engineering. Well, I came out of that 99.99 and they asked me how did I do it. Well, how do you explain seeing? How do you do that?"

They Know I Cure AIDS

↦↦↦

I once worked with a technical writer at a research and development company in Virginia. Eddie was a friendly Black man from Haiti, smart too. He moonlighted as a medical technician and didn't mind sharing all he knew about technology, science, medicine and current affairs. When he spoke with his thick French accent my ears perked up at the sound of it. I studied French from second grade through college and enjoyed refreshing what I learned with Eddie. But most of the time we talked about his science and medical background. Actually, it seemed more like classroom instructions with Eddie explaining things like gametes and bacteria.

One morning, AIDS made its way into our conversation. Eddie talked about the combination of gametes and feces—a virtual explosion in the body—creating a virus that destroys the body's immune system. In those days, the mid-80s, AIDS-related deaths crept into television news every day. Two popular African American broadcasters in Washington, D.C. succumbed to it, one of them a fellow alumnus of Howard University's School of Communications.

ॐ ॐ ॐ

Melvin Lindsey's smooth bassy voice held radio audiences captive every weeknight from 7 p.m. to 11 p.m. when he hosted WHUR-FM's groundbreaking program *The Quiet Storm*. It catered to the lovestruck and the romantic and ranked number one in its timeslot for over eight years, with Melvin's frequent airplay of Diana Ross, Patti Austin and Luther Vandross ballads. At 7 p.m. each night, Smokey Robinson's hit song *Quiet Storm* opened the show. Like summer's warm welcome evening breeze, it flowed through speakers and into the homes and spaces of listeners dedicated to the music, dedicated to Melvin.

He was a nice guy with a quick, soft smile. If you were lucky enough to hear him laugh on one of those rare occasions, you'd hear a baritone's laugh. He was tall and caramel complexioned with a thick black curly Afro. Melvin won over the most strait-laced stoics and excelled as a student leader in the School of Communications Film Society. Who, other than Melvin, could occupy the hallowed position of number one disc jockey in Washington, D.C. all that time?

With gratitude and phenomenal heroism a few weeks before his death, Melvin allowed the broadcast of his videotaped farewell to his fans. His death in 1992 saddened all of us in the Greater Washington Metropolitan area.

When Melvin and I were students at Howard, Max Robinson advanced to the position of first Black anchor of a national newscast. ABC Television's Roone Arledge tapped him for the position after watching his meteoric rise as co-anchor on WTOP's evening news in Washington, D.C.

Robinson was a good looking virile broadcaster. He wore a thick Afro and thick moustache. But I focused on his deep resonating delivery and professional demeanor, unaware of the career battles he waged off camera. The title "first Black" has its obstacles, Robinson once stated. He died of AIDS December 20, 1988, after delivering a physically taxing speech at Howard University's School of Communications. The Max Robinson Center at the Whitman-Walker AIDS Clinic of Washington, D.C. is named in his honor.

かかか

I shared Eddie's information with Dr. Sebi. He admitted he didn't know what Eddie knew. He knew that if AIDS attacked the immune system, he could rebuild the body's cells there, with the same success as all of his other AIDS clients.

"When the man told me he was cured of AIDS, I wasn't excited. And I wasn't surprised and I wasn't like, wow, I cured AIDS fellows. I told the man thank you and I went about my business. No one on the planet has proof for the cure of AIDS but me. They know that I'm curing AIDS."

If that's true, I thought, why a persistent global focus on getting tested and taking antiviral medications, instead of rebuilding body cells and diet change?

"So what is going on?" he asked. "Where is this thing?"

His cooperative mood shifted when he recalled the time he travelled to Washington, D.C. to share his expertise in combating AIDS. He accompanied singer Michael Jackson—his client at the time—to an AIDS meeting hosted by Texas Congresswoman Sheila Jackson Lee. Some of the members of the U.S. House of Representatives' Congressional Black Caucus and several African leaders attended the meeting with Michael Jackson (the invited guest and the focus of a global AIDS fundraising tour).

"I'm quite sure that the 17 African ambassadors that were present at the Rayburn Building on March 31, 2004, that they heard Dr. Sebi and they saw the document that he cures AIDS. Well, Dr. Sebi came to the conclusion that they are not interested. And that may be a good thing. Let the African people die maybe that gives way to more people coming onto the planet. Maybe that's a good thing. Maybe I'm the intruder. I'm the one that is violating their secret arrangements."

A secret arrangement to keep AIDS deaths escalating? That I couldn't fathom. The United States has contributed well over $3 billion for AIDS research and treatments. At least 6 U.S. agencies, including the Office of Minority Health, provide grants to programs and nonprofit organizations that address HIV/AIDS treatment, prevention, education and research. It could be that Dr. Sebi's prescriptions—remove poisons, rebuild the body's cells, encourage alkaline foods—met up with a bit of indifference and doubt from leaders seeking immediate, well-known remedies to the epidemic.

It wouldn't be the first time he faced the government's scrutiny. In 1988, a few months shy of the first World AIDS Day, the New York Supreme Court acquitted Dr. Sebi—Alfredo Bowman is his legal name—of false advertising in New York City newspapers. He claimed he could cure AIDS and advertised it. Someone alerted New York State Attorney General Robert Abrams about the advertisements. Abrams ordered the unlicensed Alfredo

Bowman to remove the ads from all newspapers. Dr. Sebi refused. He was arrested and served a brief time in jail before his trial. With testimonies from over 70 cured clients, he won his case (picking up a few new clients in the process) and continued to practice natural healing with his herbal products.

Patience, far-sightedness and great care and coordination can bridge the gap between Dr. Sebi and his skeptics.

CHAPTER 9

RELIGION GIVES WAY TO INDEPENDENCE

He is so fiercely independent that when any hint of infringement of it comes he withdraws. He retreats to the Florida Everglades or Key West or Usha Village. He'll drive from Los Angeles, California down to Central America, stopping only for gasoline or plant watching. It's a freedom conceived in his life with Mama Hay.

Between 2004 and 2005, Dr. Sebi dictated his autobiography, giving it the title *The Cure: The Autobiography of Dr. Sebi "Mama Hay."* He named it in honor of his grandmother whose birth name was Ann, but the community where she read tarot cards called her Mama Hay.

Dr. Sebi weaved stories of a strong Haitian woman into our conversations, telling me that more than anything else Mama Hay taught him impenetrable self-reliance. She sent young Alfredo to a Christian church, but independence influenced her behavior. She had embraced the teachings of early 20th century Black movement leader Marcus Garvey and those, more than Christianity, shaped the mindset she passed onto her grandson.

Garvey was a Jamaican man who built an ocean liner to transport willing African descendants back to Africa, an idea postured by his group, the Universal Negro Improvement Association (UNIA). Organized in 1917, UNIA members operated grocery stores, laundries and restaurants. They owned printing plants, clothing factories and the steamship line. It was the first Black mass movement with 700 branches in 38 states and the West Indies, and as of this writing continues the work of its founder. Dr. Sebi speaks often at UNIA conferences.

Neither Mama Hay nor Dr. Sebi travelled on Garvey's ocean liner back to Africa. Dr. Sebi would travel there many times on his own. But from that rock solid spirit of self-preservation, Usha Village, the Usha Research Institute, and Dr. Sebi the healer were realized.

I noticed mild constraint when he mentioned the millions of dollars he declined from an investor that requested his products' formula in exchange for his investment in the Usha Research Institute.

I saw Usha Village as a work-in-progress and considered that multimillion dollar investment a boost to upgrading it. Air conditioning or ceiling fans replacing table fans; an emergency generator for blackouts; a landscaped meditation trail running from the cabins down to the hot spring and into the rainforest. But I understood Dr. Sebi's decision. He held fast to two of the strongest symbols of his independence—Usha Research Institute and her formula. Any changes to Usha Village would come by his own means.

Conversations about Marcus Garvey and self-preservation ushered in the announcement he converted to the Islamic faith and joined the Nation of Islam. I couldn't see the connections at first. I saw a determined healer in loose cotton attire and sandals, not a man inclined to wear a uniformed bowtie and dark suit. But he helped me see that joining the Nation of Islam was a natural progression from his life with Mama Hay.

"So what attracted you to the Nation of Islam?" I asked, caught off guard by his participation in the regimens of religion.

"What attracted me to the Nation of Islam is that I grew up in a Garvey house. And growing up in a Garvey house you get this pride, this sense of value that you add to yourself. So I automatically took on that particular persona because my grandmother was one hell of a Black woman. She was uncompromising. She didn't care how big or how small you were. In her eyes you were the same. But she had this sense of value about herself that I seldom see in people. So when I came to America, coming from this house of Garvey, well yes, independence is the thing of the day. Sure I was happy when I heard about the messenger Elijah Muhammad was going to construct schools, farms, hospitals. Well naturally, fresh out of a Garvey house, I am attracted to this. It's a magnet now, you know, there's affinity, and I love it. I love Malcolm. I love Elijah and I sit at the table at South Woodlawn Avenue in Chicago at Messenger Elijah Muhammad's house and sat and ate with the Holy Apostle. All of our brothers, all of our brothers and sisters that came to us, came to us with different givings, to suffice different areas of our journey."

"What made you go to the Nation of Islam meeting?"

"When I got to New Orleans I got hooked up with the barbershop, Tim's Barbershop, because I liked the energy there. And these brothers were the ones who introduced me to Islam. They were talking this strong thing that I associated with Garvey."

And after three decades of separation from the Nation of Islam Dr. Sebi feels just as beholden to the group as he does Mama Hay's blueprint for self-preservation.

"When I was in the Nation of Islam I loved the Nation of Islam. I love the Nation of Islam now, and I will always love the Nation of Islam because what I received in the Nation of Islam I could only have received it in the Nation of Islam. There were components that the Nation of Islam offered that the other entities, religious or philosophical, did not have to offer. But it was offered in the Nation of Islam. At the time that I was a Muslim, it was in the middle 1950s. Then, it was a different air about the brothers. We were happy and the community loved us. The Christian community loved us in New Orleans and we loved the Christian community. We even bought a vegetable truck to bring them fresh vegetables every day. We would pick up their clothes because the Christians were the ones that gave us their business, you understand. So I cannot see why there should not be love among the Christians and the Muslims because as you know, as you and I both know, if I love Muslims and Christians, hey, that's beautiful, it makes it easy for me."

Only fitness guru Jack LaLanne rivals his youthful vigor and commitment to life. He revamped his energy and his lifestyle, almost cold turkey it seemed, not gradual like mine.

"When you were sick with asthma and the other diseases, what were you doing?" I asked him.

"The same as everyone else. I ate meat. I ate chicken. I ate everything. The Christians told me it's good to eat hogs. The Muslims say it's good to eat lamb. But as I ingested these foods recommended by these religions, which I was a member of, my body remained sick. It was sicker, every day getting worse. And one day, I went to Mexico with the recommendation from the brother from New Orleans. The Mexican said are you ready to be healed? He said, 'Now you are going to listen to me. I will remove the food that God did not make or is not supposed to be in your mouth.' That was 42 years ago and I'm happy as a lark."

"That's what we should do?"

"We could violate God if we want to. My brother did. If I want to violate God, well, it's up to me. I violate God, who's going to pay? I'm going to pay. My brother paid with his life but he didn't care."

"Your brother that was a reverend?"

"My brother that was a reverend." He speaks of his late half-brother Felix Gale.

"He preached for many, many, many years. Good man here in La Ceiba. That's right at the same place you go last night, the town. But my brother, like many other pastors, are not to be blamed for not going to the medicine of the very God they preach about. They were unaware of the devastating impact that glucose would have on the hypothalamus. They were totally unaware. So yes, they love God and they preach God. But they were doing something a little bit different. Because when they get sick, they

went to a chemical. That's telling God, God I hear you but I can't do it. We have to make ourselves aware, hey, look, where are we going with this thing? Look at the rate of murders. Look at the rate of mothers killing their children, one of the things that's un- heard of. A mother killing her child? She has to kill. She has to kill her children. Why? She's been compelled to do that."

Yet another jolt. "Why do you say compelled?"

"Because she's eating the things that precipitate that. Yeast will cause you to disrupt things. But if there's peace, man, money could come later. You know, I'm chillin'."

"Sleep well," I chimed in.

"But to chill you can't eat a hot dog and say I'm chillin' because I know what that hot dog is going to do. The uric acid is going to play havoc on our what? The central nervous system. But our children are saying, 'Man, I'm chillin'.' But look, it's like the guru and the Dalai Lama. They be telling us about peace, about what we need to do about peace, how to obtain peace. They tell us, right? But when you go home to eat, the very thing you put in your mouth undermines the goal you're pursuing. So that's why I was never impressed with either one."

"I see. It makes perfect sense."

"But if the Dalai Lama's message was nutrition, he wouldn't need to talk to people because in the state of health is where the brain is reconnecting to the cosmic procession. The thing that you should see, you will see those things. And they are not in any book. Because I just showed you one. The curing of the lady, putting the substance on her head. That doesn't come out of a book. It came out of Sebi."

A village called Utopia couldn't have crowned a wiser sire. Relaxed, unpretentious, confident with his asser- tions—all tried and true. I agree that it's difficult to define or explain cosmic arrangements or vibrations. You live it. I felt it then, serenity, slow easy breaths and a gentle move back on the futon's pillows. My eyes settled, no folds in my forehead, only peace, inner, outward, Dr. Sebi's word—cosmic.

Brothers and sisters when you go
back to where you came from, England, America,
the Caribbean, don't you ever put starch in your mouth
again. Don't do it. Begin to wean yourself, gradually. I'm
not asking you to make a cold turkey change. Don't do it.
But you will gradually, in increments, in degrees, right?
And one day when you're over here, you'll say
I feel good, you know. I feel good.

**–Dr. Sebi Speaks to Visitors at
Usha Village, September 20, 2008**

Chapter 10

Free Flowing

It takes me one hour to walk a one-mile loop around a Palos Verdes neighborhood that overlooks the Pacific Ocean. Sometimes it takes longer. When honeysuckle and rose bushes invite me to slow down and take a whiff, I accept. I stroke the tip of birds of paradise and wink at palms hugging entranceways and windows. The views are serene and absolutely breathtaking. Landscaped front lawns at stuccoed bungalows and two-story Cape Cods; Mediterranean-style haciendas with sweeping views of the Pacific.

Breathing in, I savor it. Breathing out, I adore it. My body supplies ample energy, ample oxygen for these meditative and therapeutic walks. But as an asthmatic, my lungs constricting with every step, my mini tour wouldn't last ten minutes.

The desensitization shots I received in my childhood helped me with my allergies. But Dr. Sebi's admonitions alerted me that clear lungs and good health require more effort and a willingness to return to the natural. The alarm went off and floodgates of information burst open with real food alternatives.

I've created at least five ways to cook a new staple in my kitchen—chickpeas, that underrated legume chock full of fiber, calcium, iron, magnesium, phosphorous, potassium and vitamin A. I'm not a full-fledged vegetarian—yet. I love seafood, a frequent dish my spelt penne pasta and broiled shrimp, the deveined shrimp marinated overnight in sea salt and onion powder. With this dish I'll have chickpea patties (chickpea steaks if you prefer a gourmet description) and either green beans or asparagus. There's fish on the plate but the meal is far more alkaline than acidic.

There's a global need to shift from inexpensive bulk starch-based stimulants, as Dr. Sebi calls them, to economical life-sustaining alkaline food, food that energizes the body and replenishes all the good converted things that come out in our waste. Iron out, iron in. Fiber out, fiber in. Vitamins A through K out, vitamins A through K in. Potassium out, potassium in. Alkaline out, alkaline in.

And should the majority of us heal and live healthy lives, there will still be a need for doctors. Yes, as long as we all love to run, jump, climb, do daredevil stunts, as long as we monitor our health from time to time with checkups, doctors remain a viable part of our society.

My purpose in life is to learn and be happy. . . . Yes, I am vegetarian.

–Sting

APPENDIX

Food Guide—An Introduction

࿇࿇࿇

Health food bland and tasteless? Prepared with the right seasonings and patient creativity, natural foods debunk the myth that health foods leave you wanting for something weighty and, yes, meaty.

For dinner tonight may I suggest mashed chickpeas, gravy and onions, green beans, mushroom patties and a garden salad with cucumber dressing? And for breakfast tomorrow morning I recommend Portobello mushroom bacon, spelt bread toast with mango jam or maple butter and homemade apple sauce sweetened with 100% maple syrup. I prefer Grade A Dark Amber.

The options are endless. All it takes is patient substitution and weaning, and the following food guide and recipes to get you started.

Reconnecting with Dr. Sebi opened the door to some fantastic ways to prepare not only delicious healthy foods, but delicious comfort foods, many reminiscent of my childhood. For instance, if you like the taste of fried chicken gizzards and livers, for a healthy alternative you can replace the chicken with oyster mushrooms, season them with olive oil, sea salt, kelp, cayenne pepper and chickpea (also called garbanzo bean) flour and fry or broil them in the oven. You can replace boiled potatoes with stewed chickpeas and onions. I like them seasoned with sea salt, curry powder and just a pinch of cayenne pepper. And my new cherished seasonings are onion powder and onion sea salt—two great replacements for garlic, which has a pH value below 3.

Some of the vegetables in the food guide were new to me when Dr. Sebi introduced them. They were Latin-oriented, reflecting Dr. Sebi's Spanish origins: agave nectar (natural sweetener), tomatillos, nopales and izote (cactus vegetables). With the food revolution going on now, you can purchase these products not only in Latin Markets but in large health food stores.

You're thinking, "I've been to health food stores. The food prices are sky high. I have a family of five to feed," or "My monthly social security benefits and pension won't allow me to buy high priced health food," or "In my retirement planning I didn't factor in spending $5 for a loaf of spelt bread or $10 for a bottle of maple syrup." Points well taken and understood. I suppose the rules of supply and demand apply here. When more people catch onto and buy healthy tasty food products, prices will fall. They must. Our organs and immune system demand it.

I'm not advocating we replace traditional grocery stores with health food stores. Traditional grocers in the United States—Vons, Ralphs, Pathmark, Safeway, Giant, Kroger—have heeded a call for natural and organic foods. I was grocery shopping one afternoon and was surprised when I found pre-sliced Portobello mu- 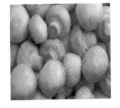 shrooms on a display of mushrooms that must have spanned three feet wide. Oyster mushrooms, button, Portobello, all beautifully arranged. And at that same store I pulled my almond milk from the shelf.

No need to put anyone out of work, just a shift in food production and availability. Cow milk farmers could shift to buffalo (natural animal) milk farming. Peanut growers could shift to almonds. Chickpea fries are the new French fry. And speaking of shifting, here's a food challenge. Calling all cake bakers — mothers, grandmothers, godmothers, aunts, sisters, fathers. Try shifting **from** salt, sugar, milk, eggs, white flour, and cake flour **to** sea salt, maple sugar, buffalo or almond milk, spelt flour and egg replacer. Now there's a show I'd watch on a food channel.

And lest we forget — fast foods. What to do about them?

Even after a decision is made to buy and eat healthy natural foods, the time will come (speaking from experience here) when you tire of preparing it every night and will seek pre-cooked meals outside the home.

You're thinking, "Health food stores sell frozen health foods, Beverly," or "Coffee shops and delis sell vegetarian sandwiches and soups." All true points. But rarely is the sandwich made with spelt, rye, or kamut bread or non-dairy almond cheese. And soups are seasoned — under the guise of spices — with black pepper, a carcinogen known to cause inflammation of the skin and to cause adverse effects on reproductive organs and the gastrointestinal tract. Even Jethro Kloss, in his bestselling book *Back to Eden*, recommends cayenne pepper instead of black pepper.

Calling all budding fast food entrepreneurs. Who will give us an order of chickpea fries or chickpea fritters to go? Chickpea battered onion rings? Vanilla almond milkshake with a donut made with spelt, chopped almonds and maple sugar? Or crispy vegetable rolls filled with greens?

Now on to the food guide, suggested by Dr. Sebi.

FRUITS

APPLES: origin—Asia, as sour apples; ancient Romans grafted apples to yield a variety; by Stone Age they spread over much of Europe **nutritional value**—vitamins A and C; low in fat; rich in cellulose; aids digestion.

APRICOTS: origin—Ancient China; spread to Greece and Rome; by 17th century reached the Americas **nutritional value**—rich in vitamins A and C, fiber and potassium; eaten as dried fruit, jam or fresh fruit.

BANANAS (classified as a large berry): origin—Asia; Arabs carried them to Near East and the Mediterranean; travelled to the Caribbean and Mexico in the 15th century **nutritional value**—good source of vitamins A and C and potassium; they do not contain starch like the larger green plantains; plantains lose starch and become sweeter, banana-like when they turn yellow.

BERRIES (blueberries): origin—grow wild in Scandinavia, British Isles, North and South America; cross-bred in United States in 1909 **nutritional value**—vitamin C; **(blackberries and raspberries): origin**—native to Asia, Europe, North America; grows wild; two commercial type raspberries, red and black; many blackberry varieties, including boysenberry, black pearl, and dewberry **nutritional value**—vitamin C; low in calories; **(cranberries): origin**—native and grow wild in Northeast United States **nutritional value**—high in vitamin C.

CHERRIES: origin—date back to pre-historic times, native to Asia Minor; found in Stone Age European caves and cliff dwellings in America **nutritional value**—good source of vitamins A and C.

COCONUTS: origin—pre-historic tropical fruit of palm trees native to the Tropics, including Polynesia, Hawaii, Malaysia **nutritional value**—good source of dietary fiber, iron and potassium.

CURRANTS: origin—native to ancient Greece; grow wild in temperate to subarctic regions, including England, Germany and Scandinavia **nutritional value**—considered raisin grape, these tiny scarlet berries are also black or white; high in vitamin C, potassium and fiber.

DATES: origin—native to Nile Valley as early as 3500 B.C.; grow well in arid areas; often considered the "candy that grows on trees" **nutritional value**—good source of calcium and B complex; date honey made from juice of the fruit.

FIGS: origin—Western Asia and the Mediterranean Basin, one of the most ancient fruits used and revered by Greeks and Romans; Spanish explorers introduced them to America **nutritional value**—high in dietary fiber; good source of iron and calcium.

GRAPES (with seeds): origin—ancient vine fruits; exact origins unknown; found in ancient Greek and Roman murals and mosaics; growing wild in Northeast North America in pre-Columbian times **nutritional value**—potassium, vitamin C, natural sugars.

LIMES (key limes): origin—Mexican limes now grown in Florida, smaller, rounder than Persian or Bearss limes **nutritional value**—high in vitamin C; processed into juice and sold for use in key lime pie; also used in salads, seafood.

MANGOES: origin—native of India and the Himalayan region; grown for over 6,000 years; North American mangoes grown primarily in Florida and Mexico **nutritional value**—high in vitamins A and C, fiber and potassium.

MELONS including cantaloupes: origin—Persia; spread to Europe over 3,000 years ago; arrived in Americas in the 15th century **nutritional value**—high in vitamins A and C.

ORANGES: origin—native to Asia; spread to Near East and North Africa in the 9th century, Spain and Portugal in the 12th, by the 16th century flourished in North and South America **nutritional value**—high in vitamins A, C, and potassium.

PAPAYAS: origin—the Americas and Mexico; brought to Hawaii by Spanish settlers **nutritional value**—high in vitamins A and C; smooth flesh similar to melons; sweet pulp high in potassium; good source of fiber.

PASSION FRUIT: origin—Brazil; purple fruit thrives in temperate climates; the yellow fruit in tropical and subtropical climates **nutritional value**—tropical fragrance tart fruit.

PEACHES: origin—wild fruit native to China as far back as 5 B.C.; spread to Near East and Greece and Rome; in Persia called Persian plum or Persian apple; introduced to North America by Christopher Columbus **nutritional value**—high in vitamins A and C.

PEARS: origin—Ancient Greece and Rome, were only grown in gardens of castles and monasteries; arrived in American colonies in the 17th century; noted varieties anjou, bosc, bartlett **nutritional value**—good source of vitamins A and C and fiber.

PINEAPPLES: origin—native to pre-Incas of Peru; introduced to Christopher Columbus in the 15th century by Indians; explorers and traders spread fruit throughout Africa and the tropics, including the Philippines and Hawaii **nutritional value**—high in vitamin C and fiber.

PLUMS: origin—ancient fruit native to temperate climate areas worldwide; gathered by Stone Age tribes; spread to Mediterranean region; introduced to Japan 300 years ago **nutritional value**—high in potassium; contains calcium, iron and vitamin C.

POMEGRANATES: origin—Ancient Persia, Near East; staple fruit in Eastern and Mediterranean countries **nutritional value**—sweet and tart flavored fruit of seeds wrapped in juicy pulp; high in potassium.

PRUNES: origin—plum species (see above) dried chewy fruit **nutritional value**—good source of vitamin A, dietary fiber, potassium, copper.

SOURSOPS: origin—pre-Columbian Mexico, Central and South America, sub-Saharan Africa **nutritional value**—tropical fruit, pulp is like pineapple; good source of calcium and phosphorous.

STRAWBERRIES: origin—grow wild on many continents; colonists saw them in North America in the 17th century **nutritional value**—high in vitamin C, iron and other minerals.

SUGAR APPLES: origin—Tropical Americas, India, Pakistan; cultivated in the Caribbean, Florida, the tropics **nutritional value**—tropical sweet fruit, flesh tastes like custard, sweet-smelling fragrance; good source of iron and calcium.

VEGETABLES

ASPARAGUS: origin—ancient grass as far back as 200 B.C.; native to Eastern Mediterranean where it grows wild; member of the lily of the valley family **nutritional value**—high in vitamins A and C and potassium.

AVOCADOES (ahuacatl, hardy Fuerte): origin—native to Mexico and Guatemala 3 B.C.; spread to South America where it was cultivated by the Aztecs and Incas **nutritional value**—good source of vitamins A, C, and E, iron and potassium.

BELL PEPPERS or sweet peppers: origin—South America 5000 B.C.; carried throughout world by Spanish explorers **nutritional value**—high in vitamins A and C, small amounts of calcium, phosphorous, iron, magnesium.

CHICKPEAS (garbanzo): origin—Middle East 7000 B.C.; cultivated in the Mediterranean Basin beginning 3000 B.C. **nutritional value**—a legume high in dietary fiber, iron, folate, copper, manganese.

COLLARD GREENS: origin—Asia Minor, Celtic groups in 600 B.C. introduced plant to Europe; spread to America in the 17th century **nutritional value**—member of the wild cabbage family; excellent source of vitamins A, C, K and E, B-complex vitamins; good antioxidant; high in calcium, potassium, iron, phosphorous; contain sulfur-based phytonutrients. (Recommended by author)

CUCUMBERS: origin—Asia, between the Bay of Bengal and the Himalayas over 5,000 years ago; found in ancient Egypt, Greece and Rome **nutritional value**—low in calories; small amounts of vitamins and minerals; slicing and pickling varieties available year round.

DANDELION GREENS: origin—grow wild throughout Asia, Europe and North America; long leaf, deep notch leaves, weed of the chicory family; in colonial America used as a spring tonic; commercial varieties less bitter than wild dandelions **nutritional value**—good source of vitamins A and C, iron, calcium and riboflavin.

EGGPLANT: origin—Asia; brought to Turkey, Greece, Spain and Italy by Arab traders; brought to the New World by Spanish explorers; bright colored varieties, including white, gray, green; called Aubergine in Europe **nutritional value**—good source of potassium and fiber.

IZOTE (cactus flower): origin—pre-Columbian Central America and Mexico; national flower of El Salvador **nutritional value**—edible flowering plant cooked in Latin dish pupusa or scrambled with other foods.

KALE: origin—ancient Greece and Rome; chief winter vegetable for England for over 1,000 years **nutritional value**—large hardy curly leaves; good source of vitamins A and C, iron and calcium.

LETTUCE: origin—ancient Asia Minor; wild in the Mediterranean areas by the Middle Ages; the first garden vegetable in the American colonies **nutritional value**—the greener the leaves, the richer the source of vitamins A, C, and E, as well as iron, calcium and other minerals.

MUSHROOMS: origin—Egyptian Pharaohs declared them sacred; Romans called them food of the Gods but allowed everyone to eat them on holy days and holidays; commercially grown varieties are of the single species *Agaricus campestris* **nutritional value**—good source of B-complex vitamins; high in minerals, especially iron and copper.

MUSTARD GREENS: origin—also known as Indian mustard in reference to origins in India; mustard seed comes from this plant; 2,000 years ago Romans used them to cure epilepsy, lethargy and pains of the day **nutritional value**—good source of vitamins A and C.

NOPALES: origin—Mexico **nutritional value**—when cooked, soft but crunchy; flavor of green pepper, string beans and asparagus; good source of vitamins A, B and C, and iron.

OKRA: origin—Africa; also known as okro, gombo, ochro, quia-bo; grows wild in Africa today as in prehistoric times; grows in climates with long hot summers **nutritional value**—tender, sweet, slippery when cooked; high in vitamins A and C, calcium, potassium.

OLIVES: origin—7000 B.C. in coastal areas of the Mediterranean Basin, including Southwestern Europe, Northern Africa, Western Asia; grown farther inland today; classified as a fruit and sacred plant **nutritional value**—good source of antioxidant vitamin E, also iron, copper and dietary fiber.

ONIONS: origin—prehistoric Asia Minor "the Fertile Crescent"; Egyptians used them as food, medicine and symbol of the Universe and eternity; used extensively by ancient Greeks and Romans **nutritional value**—flavor value more prominent than nutritional value; 38 calories in medium-sized onion; low in sodium.

PUMPKIN: origin—Mexico and North America 5500 B.C.; staple in American Indian meals, seeds as well; spread throughout Europe by explorers **nutritional value**—good source of zinc, phosphorous, magnesium, copper and vitamin K.

SEA VEGETABLES/SEAWEED: origin—the sea; ancient use native to Japan; green, brown, red and blue-green algae **nutritional value**—bladderwrack (vitamin K, adrenal stimulant); dulse (rich in iron, protein, vitamin A); kelp (vitamins A, B, C, D and K, rich in minerals, can be purchased as a food seasoning); nori (sweet, meaty taste when dried, used as a sushi wrapper, rich in protein, fiber, calcium, iron, phosphorous, can be purchased as a dry snack).

SPINACH: origin—Persia (now Iran); brought to Europe by the Moors; smooth leaf spinach and crumpled leaf spinach **nutritional value**—contains vitamins A, B and C and iron; also contains natural oxalic acid.

SQUASH (including butternut squash): origin—North America 5000 B.C.; called askootasquash by American Indians; relative of gourds and pumpkins **nutritional value**—low in sodium, high in vitamins A and C; three basic classifications: soft-shelled, small, immature; hard-shelled, mature, small; and hard-shelled, mature, large.

STRING BEANS: origin—Peru; spread to South and Central America by migrating Indian tribes; introduced to Europe around the 16th century by Spanish explorers **nutritional value**—high in vitamins A, C and K; good source of magnesium, thiamin, copper, calcium, phosphorous.

TOMATILLOS: origin—Aztec; primarily grown in Mexico and southern California; also known as Mexican green tomato, tomate verde; widely used in Mexican salsas; also called Chinese lantern plants because fruits are enclosed in papery calyxes that cover them like oriental lampshades; tomatillos resemble green cherry tomatoes **nutritional value**—rich in vitamins A and C, and niacin; cooked primarily in sauces and dressings.

TOMATOES: origin—Mexico, called tomatl; taken to Europe by Italian explorers; was first yellow then red when it arrived in Europe; called pomo d'oro by Italians; not considered food in the United States until mid-19th century; commercial American crop in 1880s **nutritional value**—rich in vitamin C and minerals but when cooked vitamin C is reduced.

TURNIP GREENS (turnip tops, turnip salad): origin—Russia, Rome, Scandinavia; early American colonists used them as food in the 17th century **nutritional value**—not a good salad green due to bitterness and chewy toughness; best if cooked with kale, mustards and other greens; rich in vitamin A.

ZUCCHINI: origin—a variety of squash or Italian squash, also known as summer squash **nutritional value** vitamin A, potassium and manganese.

NOTE: Notice that potatoes, cassava, yams and other starch-based tuberous root vegetables are omitted from this food guide, and, according to Dr. Sebi, should be minimized or avoided. But research shows that sweet potatoes, a member of the Morning Glory family and unrelated to the yam, are rich in vitamins A, C, B6, copper, potassium and dietary fiber and do not contain the toxin dioscorine. Yams, a crop introduced to Africa and South America by Portuguese traders, contain dioscorine.

SPICES & SEASONINGS

MILD FLAVORS

Basil
Bay Leaf
Dill
Marjoram

Oregano
Savory
Tarragon
Thyme

PUNGENT & SPICY FLAVORS

Achiote
Cayenne Pepper
Coriander
Cumin

Curry
Ginger
Onion Powder

SALTY FLAVORS

Onion Sea Salt
Pure Sea Salt

Seaweed (Dry)
(kelp/dulse/nori)

SWEET FLAVORS

Agave Nectar
Date Sugar
(dried dates)

100% Maple Syrup
Maple Sugar
(dried maple syrup)

GRAINS

Amaranth	Spelt
Kamut	Tef
Quinoa	Wild Rice
Rye	

These natural grains can be found in major health food stores in the form of breads, cereals, flours, and pasta.

NUTS & SEEDS

Almonds	Pumpkin Seeds
Almond Butter	Sesame Seeds
Brazil Nuts	Sesame Tahini
*Pecans	Walnuts

HERBAL TEAS

Allspice	Fennel
Anise	Ginger
Chamomile	Lemongrass
Natural Mint	

*While high in healthy fat (72%), pecans are also high in manganese (an antioxidant), as well as iron, vitamin B6, vitamin E, potassium, calcium and phosphorous.

MEDICINAL HERBS
(A FEW RECOMMENDED BY DR. SEBI)

BLADDERWRACK: a form of kelp; good source of iodine, calcium, magnesium, potassium, iron, sulfur and B-complex vitamins; relieves constipation, good for thyroid problems, including hypothyroidism; relieves heartburn, rheumatism and rheumatoid arthritis.

BLUE VERVAIN: a North American perennial herb; edible and medicinal, especially in early American Indian culture; leaves and roots used as a remedy for ulcers, headaches, bowel problems and rheumatism.

BURDOCK: a wild plant native to Europe and Northern Asia, now widespread in the United States; fresh or dried roots are used, seeds are edible; used as a blood purifier, relieves boils, rheumatism and skin disorders.

CHAMOMILE: a mild relaxant and sleeping aid; used medicinally in ancient Egypt, Greece and Rome; its popularity grew in the Middle Ages as a remedy for asthma, colic, fevers, cancer.

CHAPARRAL: native to California, Northern Baja, California and Mexico; has analgesic and antiflammatory properties; high in antioxidants; a blood purifier; relieves tumor growth.

DANDELION: high in vitamins A, C, D and B-complex vitamins, iron, magnesium and zinc; leaves and root used as a diuretic and laxative; stimulates digestion; a good blood purifier; used by Arabian physicians in the 10th and 11th centuries.

SEA MOSS: a seaweed or red algae, native to Europe and the United States; contains iodine, bromine, iron, sulfur and vitamins A and E.

YELLOW DOCK: a perennial herb indigenous to Europe and some parts of Asia, now found in the United States; fresh leaves are used in salads; the root is used as a laxative and astringent; relieves poor digestion and liver problems also swelling of nasal passages; cleanses toxins from the body.

Recipes—An Introduction

❧ ❧ ❧

On the road to right healing and right health I learned a diet high in alkaline food is the best to energize the body and prevent ill health. Moderation is key with most things in life but with diet, 80/20 is best: 80% alkaline food (natural), 20% acid (comfort foods that our taste buds crave).

Like most recipes, those on the following pages can transform into custom-made meals. Vary the seasonings (natural and alkaline) according to your taste. George Washington Carver set a precedent with over 100 uses for the peanut, a starchy food but made quite phenomenal in Mr. Carver's inventions. Now there's the almond, natural, alkaline, delicious, rich in vitamin E. Try almond mozzarella cheese on your next grilled cheese sandwich. For your milkshake, try almond milk.

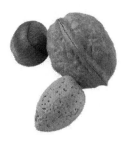

The chickpea is another versatile food that will surprise your family with all the ways you can use it. Chickpea flour can be used as gravy mix and a nutritious alternative batter.

As I said earlier, alkaline options are endless. Remember spelt? In addition to bread, spelt growers use the grain to make spelt elbow macaroni and spelt lasagna noodles. And how about spelt penne and rotini pastas? You'll find all these in most health food stores and on the Internet. Without further adieu—**The Recipes.**

Breakfast

Banana Breakfast Shake

2 cups of vanilla almond milk or coconut milk
1 medium banana
½ cup of maple syrup or agave nectar

Blend water, banana, milk and maple syrup. Blend until smooth then serve.

Crunchy Almond Butter and Strawberry Jam Sandwich

2 slices of spelt bread
*Crunchy almond butter
Strawberry jam

Toast spelt bread to desired taste. Spread almond butter on both slices. Add strawberry jam.

*Some brands have almond butter only. Other brands add sea salt. Feel free to add your own sea salt for added taste.

Kamut Puff Cereal (Cold)

Organic Kamut Puffs
Cold almond milk or coconut milk
Maple sugar

Prepare cereal the same way you would prepare other cold milk cereals. Add desired amount of kamut puffs in bowl. Cover with desired amount of cold almond or coconut milk. Sweeten with maple sugar or maple syrup.

NOTE: For thicker milk, mix sliced banana and milk in a blender.

Kamut Puff Cereal (Hot)

2 cups of vanilla almond milk or coconut milk
1 ½ cup of kamut puffs
½ cup of maple crystals
½ tsp. of cinnamon

Add milk to a pot and bring to a boil. After boiling remove pot from stove. Add kamut puffs to milk and mix until thick. Add maple crystals and cinnamon. Stir then serve.

Portobello Mushroom Bacon

1 Portobello mushroom thinly sliced, discard stem
¼ cup olive oil
Dash of sea salt
Dash of onion powder
Dash of cayenne pepper (optional)
½ cup chickpea flour or spelt flour

Coat sliced mushroom with olive oil, save remaining oil for cooking. Season mushroom slices with sea salt, onion powder and cayenne pepper. Coat mushroom with flour (optional). Heat olive oil in skillet until hot. Place slices in oil and cook each side until medium to dark brown.

Spelt French Toast

2 slices of spelt bread
1 cup of almond milk
2 tsp. of quinoa flakes
2 tsp. of spelt flour
2 tsp. of maple crystals
¼ tsp. of sea salt

Mix milk, flakes, flour, crystals and sea salt. Dip bread in mixture until coated but not soggy. Add olive oil to pan to lightly fry slices on both sides.

Spelt Toast and Mango Jam

2 slices of spelt bread
Mango jam or preserves
Non-dairy, non-soy butter or magarine (optional)

Toast bread to desired taste. Spread butter on both slices.
Spread each slice with mango jam or preserves.

Toasted Almond Mozzarella Cheese, Mushroom and Onion Sandwich

2 slices of spelt bread
1 slice of almond mozzarella cheese
1 small sweet onion
1 cap of Portobello mushroom
1 Tbs. Olive oil
Sea salt (optional)
Cayenne pepper (optional)

Slice mushroom and onion lengthwise and about 1/8 inch thick. Use just enough of the combined veggies to cover your bread. Heat olive oil in pan on medium. Toast spelt bread to desired taste. While bread toasts, sauté mushroom and onion in olive oil until onion is translucent and mushroom is tender. Sprinkle with sea salt and cayenne pepper if you prefer. Top mixture with cheese and continue to cook until cheese starts to melt. Use a spatula to remove mixture from pan and onto toast.

NOTE: You can also prepare this meal like a grilled cheese sandwich, grilling the non-dairy buttered bread in the pan, topping it with the sautéed mixture.

Dinner

Asparagus and Onions

½ bunch of asparagus, cut in half
½ small yellow onion
1 ½ qt. of water
1 Tbs. sea salt
¼ tsp. curry powder
Dash of cayenne pepper (optional)

Bring water to a rapid boil. Add sea salt, curry powder and cayenne pepper to boiling water. Chop onion and add to water. Continue boiling 5-10 minutes. Reduce boil to a simmer. Add asparagus and cook 3-5 minutes. Do not overcook. (steam cook if your prefer) Remove asparagus and onion from heat and serve.

Avocado Dressing

3 ripe avocados, peeled and seeded
½ small red onion
½ tomato peeled
¼ cup fresh lime juice
4 Tbs. pure olive oil
Dash cayenne pepper
Few sprigs of cilantro, chopped
½ tsp. chili powder
1 tsp. oregano
1 tsp. cumin
½ tsp. sweet basil
½ tsp. thyme
¼ tsp. sea salt
Spring water

Purée avocados in blender. Add remaining ingredients and 2 tablespoons of spring water. Lightly blend and pour over salad.

NOTE: Season to taste, use virgin olive oil.

Chickpea Patties (Falafel)

Falafel
1 pound dried chickpeas soaked in cold water in refrigerator overnight
1 small onion, coarsely chopped
1 tsp. onion powder
1Tbs. spelt flour
1 Tbs. ground coriander
1 tsp. baking soda
1 Tbs. ground cumin
Sea salt and cayenne pepper, as needed
½ cup olive oil

Drain the chickpeas and place them with the onion in the bowl of a food processor or blender. Add the rest of the ingredients, except the oil. Mix well. Process the mixture a second time. Form the mixture into walnut-sized balls and deep-fry or pan fry in hot oil.

Sandwich Ingredients
6 to 8 pitas, tops sliced open and lightly toasted
Shredded lettuce, as needed
Tomato wedges, or chopped tomato
Sliced red onion, as needed
Tahini sauce, recipe follows

Chickpea Patties (Falafel)
(continued)

Tahini Sauce
1Tbs. onion powder
1 tsp. sea salt
½ cup tahini (sesame seed paste)
½ cup water
1 lemon, juiced

Combine onion powder and sea salt. Add the tahini, mixing well. The sauce will thicken. Gradually add the water, blending thoroughly. Then add the lemon juice and blend well. See next page to complete sandwich.

Making the Sandwich
Stuff the pitas with lettuce and place the falafel patties on top or falafel then lettuce on top. Top with the rest of the sandwich ingredients and drizzle with the tahini sauce. Serve immediately.

Chickpeas (Stewed)

½ lb. dried chickpeas soaked overnight in 5-6 cups
of water in refrigerator
½ small sweet yellow onion, chopped
1Tbs. sea salt
1 tsp. curry powder
Dash of cayenne pepper
1 qt. of water

Drain water from chickpeas. Remove and discard any
chickpea skin floating in the water. In medium pot, bring
water to a rapid boil. Add onion, sea salt, curry powder and
cayenne pepper. Add chickpeas and reduce heat. Simmer
over low heat for 2 ½ to 3 hours.

NOTE: You can also make mashed chickpeas with this
recipe. After cooking, simply drain the water, keeping just
enough to make desired thickness of mashed chickpeas.

Chickpeas and Onions (Fried)

1 cup of cooked chickpeas (see note)
½ medium sweet yellow onion, sliced and halved
¼ tsp. sea salt or onion sea salt
Dash of cayenne pepper (optional)
2 Tbs. Olive oil

In large pan heat olive oil. Add onion and sauté for a minute or two. Add sea salt and chickpeas. Cook each side of mixture until the bottom of chickpeas is light brown. Stir and cook onions and chickpeas a few seconds longer, then remove and serve.

NOTE: You can use 1 cup of leftover Stewed Chickpeas from the previous recipe.

Chickpeas Soup

1 lb. dried chickpeas
½ tsp. sea salt
One 14 ½ oz. jar whole tomatoes, drained
1 cup finely chopped onion
2 Tbsp. olive oil
½ tsp. onion sea salt
1/8 tsp. cayenne pepper

In a colander rinse dried chickpeas well, then transfer to 4- or 5-quart container and cover generously with water. Cover and refrigerate overnight. The chickpeas will double or triple in size. Drain the water and put chickpeas in a heavy 5- to 6-quart pot or Dutch oven. Add 6 cups of water, keeping 1 ½ inches of water above chickpeas. Add ½ teaspoon sea salt. Simmer the chickpeas over low heat. Stir gently during cooking so chickpeas won't stick to bottom. Cook slowly for 1½ hours. Then prepare tomato sauce. Transfer drained tomatoes to a large, deep bowl and break apart with hands. Set aside. In a 12-inch skillet cook onion in hot olive oil over medium heat until soft but not brown. Add onion sea salt, cayenne pepper and tomatoes. Cook slowly, uncovered, for 5 to 10 minutes. Salt to taste if needed. Stir tomato-onion mixture into chickpeas and cook, partially covered for 30 minutes. To serve, transfer soup to individual bowls. **See Note on the next page.**

NOTE: Wait until chickpeas are slightly tender to the bite before stirring in tomato-onion mixture.

Cucumber Dressing

3 medium cucumbers, peeled
10 almonds, raw, unsalted
4 Tbs. pure olive oil
¼ cup fresh lime juice
¼ cup green onions, chopped fine
½ tsp. thyme
¼ tsp. sea salt
¼ tsp. dill
1 ½ cup spring water
Few sprigs of cilantro, chopped

Blend 10 almonds in spring water, 2 minutes on high speed. Strain and set liquid aside. Puree cucumbers in blender with almonds. Add olive oil, lime juice and remaining ingredients. Lightly blend, adding liquid, if needed. Pour over salad.

Hot Veggie Wrap

3 cups diced tomatoes
1 cup onion
1 cup diced red and green bell peppers
½ cup mushrooms, chopped
Spelt tortillas

Stir fry all vegetables for 5 minutes. Warm the spelt tortillas.
Wrap vegetables in tortillas.

$\mathcal{L}$asagna

1 red bell pepper, chopped
1 yellow onion, chopped
2 Tbs. olive oil
1 bay leaf, crumbled
1 box of spelt lasagna pasta
2 lbs. mushrooms
8 fresh tomatoes
Almond cheddar cheese
oregano, to taste
sea salt, to taste
13" deep dish baking pan

Tomato Sauce

Heat skillet and add olive oil. Place onion, bell peppers, oregano, sea salt and bay leaf in skillet and sauté. Boil tomatoes for 10 minutes. Place in ice water for 5 minutes, drain and remove skin. Blend tomato in blender (voila! fresh tomato sauce). Add tomato sauce in skillet with sautéed seasonings. Simmer for 30-45 minutes. Set aside half of sauce to be used to make Mushroom Sauce, remaining half to be used when layering. **Continued on the next page.**

Lasagna (continued)

Mushroom Sauce

Place mushrooms in water, soak 1 minute, strain and slice. Season to taste and sauté for 2 minutes, add to ½ of saved sauce, set aside for layering.

Pasta

Prepare pasta according to instructions on box. Once pasta is done, rinse with cold water for easy handling. Layer a deep baking dish with tomato sauce. Place a layer of pasta on top then a layer of mushroom sauce. Add a layer of almond cheddar cheese. Repeat steps until dish is almost full. Place 2 cups of sauce on top of remaining cheese. Bake in oven at 350 degrees for 20 minutes, until cheese is melted.

NOTE: Almond cheddar cheese can be purchased at major health food stores.

Lime & Olive Oil Dressing

¼ fresh lime, squeezed
½ cup olive oil
¼ cup spring water
1 Tbs. maple syrup
¼ tsp. sweet basil
¼ tsp. thyme
¼ tsp. oregano
¼ tsp. ground cumin

Put all ingredients in a glass bottle. Shake thoroughly and enjoy on your salad or veggie sandwich.

Mushroom Patties

2 Portobello mushrooms
¼ cup scallions
½ cup bell peppers
¼ tsp. oregano
1 pinch of cayenne pepper
¼ bunch of cilantro
1 Tbs. sea salt
1 tsp. dill
 2 tsp. onion powder
¼ cup spelt flour
olive oil for frying

Soak mushrooms for 1 minute in spring water. Remove and place in food processor with scallions and bell peppers. Add cilantro, flour and other seasonings. Mix thoroughly and form patties. Place them in heated pan with 2 Tbs. olive oil. Fry on both sides until done (approximately 3 minutes each side).

Mustard Greens & Kale Medley
(serves 10-12 people)

6 bunches of kale
6 bunches of mustard greens
½ cup olive oil
2 large red onions
¼ cup balsamic vinegar
2 tsp. sea salt
½ tsp. cayenne pepper
1 Tbs. maple sugar

Mince 2 onions and sauté in large stainless steel or ceramic pot with olive oil until tender. Add 3 bunches each of mustard greens and kale, half of the balsamic vinegar, half of the cayenne pepper, half of the sea salt and maple sugar. Sauté until greens begin to wilt. Add remaining ingredients, cover and cook on medium until greens are tender.

Spaghetti

1 box spelt spaghetti
¼ cup olive oil
2 cups of traditional marinara sauce
2 Tbs. sea salt
1 ½ Tbs. onion powder
1/8 tsp. cayenne pepper or chili powder
3 Tbs. maple syrup (medium or dark)

Cook spaghetti as directed on box. In a separate large pan,
heat olive oil. Add sea salt, onion powder, cayenne pepper
or chili powder, and maple syrup. Add traditional marina
sauce to above ingredients, stir. Cook on medium heat for
10 minutes. Stir pasta into sauce. Let stand for 5 minutes.

Spelt Penne Pasta

1 box spelt penne pasta
1 large yellow onion, chopped
*Almond mozzarella cheese
¼ cup olive oil
½ tsp. onion powder
1 tsp. sea salt
Dash of cayenne pepper
2 Tbs. organic, unrefined fresh or dried parsley

Prepare pasta according to directions on box. In a separate large pan, heat olive oil. Add onion, onion powder, sea salt, and cayenne pepper. Cook until onion is tender. Stir in pasta. Finely grate almond cheese over pasta. Stir thoroughly then add parsley. Stir again. Cook 3-5 more minutes until well blended.

Serve with salad and spelt bread.

*You can use almond cheddar cheese if you prefer it.

String Beans & Onions

1lb. of fresh string beans
½ medium sweet onion, chopped
1 ½ Tbs. sea salt
½ tsp. curry powder
 Dash of cayenne pepper
1 qt. of water

Rinse and cut string beans in half. Remove ends. Bring water to a rapid boil. Add sea salt, curry powder and cayenne pepper. Add onions and string beans. Reduce heat to medium. Cook 15-20 minutes.

String Bean Soup

1lb. of fresh string beans
½ medium sweet onion, chopped
1 Tbs. sea salt
½ Tbs. curry powder
 Dash of cayenne pepper (optional)
1 qt. of water

Rinse string beans. Cut off both ends of beans. Snap each bean in half. Bring water to a rapid boil. Add onion, sea salt, curry powder and cayenne pepper. Boil for 3-5 minutes. Add string beans then reduce heat to low. Cook for 15-20 minutes. Remove from heat and let string beans cool down a bit before placing in blender. Pour mixture into blender and puree until creamy. Serve in soup bowls and enjoy with spelt crackers or toast.

Taquitos

2 cups chopped onions
4 cups chopped mushrooms
¼ cup olive oil
1 tsp. chili powder
1 Tbs. sea salt
2 Tbs. tomato sauce
2 Tbs. oregano
2 tsp. onion powder
2 tsp. ground thyme
Soft corn shells

Heat olive oil in pan. Add onion and sauté until golden brown. Add mushroom and sauté for 5 minutes. Add remaining ingredients and stir. Wrap in corn shells tightly. Deep fry until crispy.

Wild Rice

1 box wild rice
Spring water
1 medium yellow onion, chopped fine
1 small red pepper
1 cup mushrooms (oyster or button), chopped fine
1/8 cup olive oil
1 tsp. thyme
2 tsp. oregano
1 tsp. sea salt

Soak rice in spring water overnight for best results. Cook rice according to package and set aside. Pour olive oil in hot skillet. Sauté vegetables and mushrooms 2-3 minutes. Add thyme, oregano, and sea salt. Fold in cooked rice and simmer for 20 minutes.

TIP: If you forget to soak rice overnight, parboil it for 20 minutes. Set aside loosely covered until rice opens (2-3 hours). Rinse and cook until tender.

Snacks

Apple Sauce and Maple Syrup

1 jar 23 oz. natural, no sugar added apple sauce, refrigerated
Grade A Dark Amber Maple Syrup

Place 1- to 1 ½ cups apple sauce in bowl. Add 1 teaspoon
maple syrup. Mix and enjoy a healthy alternative to ice
cream.

Kamut Puff

1 bag (6 oz.) Kamut Puffs
4 Tbsp. olive oil
1 tsp. onion sea salt

Pour Kamut Puffs in a large bowl and set aside. Heat olive oil in a sauce pan 30 seconds to 1minute. Add onion sea salt and mix. Drizzle liquid over Kamut Puffs and enjoy a delicious alternative to buttered popcorn.

Kamut Puff Granola

1 bag (6 oz.) Kamut Puffs
2.25 oz. bag almond pieces
2.25 oz. bag walnut pieces
2.25 oz. bag pecan pieces
1 cup Maple Syrup
Wax paper

In a 5- to 6-quart pot warm maple syrup over low heat. Add nuts and stir slowly into maple syrup. Remove from heat. Add Kamut Puffs. Stir mixture thoroughly, making sure all ingredients are blended well. Spread out mixture on a cookie sheet lined with wax paper. Refrigerate overnight (for best results at least 12 hours). Cut granola into 3-inch bars or break mixture into traditional granola pieces.

NOTE: Add sea salt to mixture for a salt and sweet taste.

Night Cap Banana Shake

2 cups of cold vanilla almond milk or coconut milk
½ cup of maple syrup
1/8 tsp. *Sea Moss and Bladderwrack mix
¼ cup of almond or coconut milk
1 medium banana

Mix ¼ cup of almond or coconut milk and Sea Moss and Bladderwrack mix in blender. Add maple syrup, milk and banana. Blend until smooth and serve.

*NOTE: This is the only recipe that uses a natural product made by Dr. Sebi's Office. Unlike the Breakfast Shake, the Night Cap Banana Shake is a nighttime drink because it has relaxing properties. The Sea Moss mix is high in vitamins A and vitamin B complex, zinc and calcium. It contains 92 trace minerals found in the body. It strengthens bones; curbs your appetite; dissolves fat and mucus. It's good for kidney, heart and respiratory problems.

Healthy Junk Food

Dates (with pits)
Maple Almonds
Maple Pecans
Maple Walnuts
Nori (roasted & sea salted seaweed snack)

NOTE: Nori is the same seaweed used in sushi but as a snack, it's dried, roasted and seasoned with sea salt. It tastes like thin potato chips.

BIBLIOGRAPHY

Carcione, Joe. 1972. *The Green Grocer: The Consumer's Guide to Fruits and Vegetables*. San Francisco: Chronicle Books.

Chopra, Deepak, Dean Ornish, Rustrum Roy, and Andrew Weil. 2009. "Alternative Medicine is Mainstream." *The Wall Street Journal*, http://www.online.wsj.com.

Eliasson, Anne Charlotte. 2004. *Starch in Food: Structure, Function and Applications*. Cambridge, UK: Woodhead Publishing.

Ensminger, Audrey, M. Eugene Ensminger, James E. Konlande, and John R. K. Robson. 1983. *Foods & Nutrition Encyclopedia*. Clovis, CA: Pegus Press.

Ensminger, Audrey, and MKJ Ensminger, et al. 1986. *Food for Health: A Nutrition Encyclopedia*. Clovis, CA: Pegus Press.

George Mateljan Foundation for the World's Healthiest Foods. http://www.whfoods.com.

Gooch, Ellen. "10+1 Things You May Not Know About Olive Oil." *Epikouria Magazine*, Fall/Spring 2005.

Hanh, Thich Nhat. "A Letter from Thay." October 2007, http://www.plumvillage.org.

———. 2008. "Our Environment: Touching the Gift of Life," *The Mindfulness Bell: A Journal of the Art of Mindful Living*, Spring.

———. 2007. *Power*. New York: HarperOne.

Harris, Jessica B. 1998. *The Africa Cookbook: Tastes of a Continent*. New York: Simon & Schuster.

HealthyHealing.com. "What Are Sea Vegetables?"

Kulkarni, Karmeen D. "Food, Culture, and Diabetes in the United States." *Clinical Diabetes* (2004): 190-192.

Liddell, Henry George, and Robert Scott. 1996. *A Greek-English Lexicon*. Oxford: Clarendon Press.

Maharishi Mahesh Yogi. 2001. *Science of Being and Art of Living: Transcendental Meditation*. New York: Penguin Putnam.

Mr. Showbiz Celebrity Lounge Webchat with Sting. November 1995, http://www.sting.com.

Pliny the Elder. "The Paste Used in Preparation of Paper." *Natural History*. Book XIII, Chapter 26, AD 77-79.

Schneider, Elizabeth. 1986. *Uncommon Fruits and Vegetables: A Common Sense Guide*. New York: Harper & Row.

Shibeshi, Ayalew. "Education for Rural People in Africa." UNESCO, IIEP, Addis Ababa (2005): 25.

Shook, Edward E. 1978. *An Advanced Treatise in Herbology*. Trinity Center Press.

Smith, Ifeyironwa Francisca. "The Case for Indigenous West African Food Culture." UNESCO Regional Office for Education in Africa (Senegal) (1995): 5-17.

Tina Turner, Talk at Taglich, Swiss, Swiss TV 1998.

Wood, Rebecca. 1988. *The Whole Foods Encyclopedia*. New York: Prentice-Hall.

The World Health Organization. Programmes and Projects. *Nutrition*. http://www.who.int, accessed on March 3, 2009.

INDEX

Acid, 28, 30, 95

Africa, 49, 73, 74, 84, 87, 88, 90, 92, 105, 106, 107, 108, 111, 124, 143, 144, 147, 149, 200, 201
17th and 18th centuries, 73

African American, 30, 37, 87, 103, 118, 124

Africans, 74, 88, 108

Agua Caliente, 12, 42, 54

AIDS, 55, 86, 102, 103, 105, 106, 118, 120, 121

Alfredo Bowman, 26, 41, 56, 99, 114, 120

Alkaline, 28, 30

allergies, 16

almond, 47, 92, 138, 139, 155, 159, 160, 161, 162, 164, 166, 180, 185, 196

alternative medicine, 23

antiviral medications, 106

arteries, 68

asthma, 13, 14, 16, 28, 30, 65, 77, 114, 127

babies, 66

Back to Eden, 139, *See* Jethro Kloss

beans, 134

Black Americans, 27, 56, *See* African Americans

black pepper, 139

bladderwrack, 12

blue vervain, 99

cabins, 42, 104, 124

calcium, 12, 53, 55, 66, 77, 85, 95, 100, 134, 142, 144, 145, 146, 147, 148, 196

canal, 104

Caribbean Sea, 43

carrots, 27

cassava, 71, 73, 74, 87, 110, 149

cayenne pepper, 139

Central America, 12, 25, 29, 39, 41, 43, 47, 63, 107, 123, 146, 148

Chickpeas, 77

Collard greens, 94

comfort foods, 78, 155

Community Warehouse, 25

cosmic, 29, 54, 64, 89, 97, 110, 128, 129

cure, 26, 67, 76, 102, 104, 105, 120, 121, 147

diabetes, 26, 48, 67, 76, 77, 86, 91, 92, 114

diet, 14, 21, 49, 58, 59, 78, 92,
    104, 121, 155
disease, 13, 14, 20, 56, 57, 67,
    68, 77, 78, 102, 103, 104,
    105, 114, 120
Dr. Sebi's Office, LLC, 38,
    196

education, 57, 59, 65, 117
Edward Shook, 79
endometriosis, 26
energy, 54, 86, 88, 103, 113,
    126, 127, 133
Eva Salve, 37

fast food, 75
Felix Gale, 127
flora, 42, 48
Florida Everglades, 123
food, 13, 16, 17, 25, 26, 28, 29,
    31, 48, 49, 50, 54, 63, 65, 66,
    68, 69, 71, 74, 75, 79, 84, 87,
    88, 89, 92, 93, 95, 103, 104,
    110, 117, 127, 134, 137, 138,
    139, 140, 146, 147, 148, 149,
    151, 155, 171, 180, 182

gari. See cassava
Garifuna, 73
global warming, 47
Great Migration, 18
Group Health Association,
    14

Guinea, 105

healer, 42, 50, 56, 57, 83, 101,
    124, 125
healers, 56, 105, 106
healing, 12, 13, 20, 25, 26, 29,
    40, 42, 49, 56, 58, 65, 69, 84,
    85, 86, 88, 103, 106, 109,
    111, 113, 114, 117, 120, 155
health, 13, 14, 17, 19, 20, 26,
    28, 29, 42, 48, 49, 50, 54, 58,
    67, 68, 69, 74, 75, 76, 86, 87,
    88, 95, 106, 115, 116, 128,
    134, 137, 138, 139, 151, 155,
    180
health food, 138
heart, 68
herbal, 26, 30, 38, 83, 106,
    113, 120
herbal compounds, 26
herbalist, 11, 21, 28, 29, 30,
    41, 50, 63, 65, 79, 112
herbs, 12, 25, 28, 29, 40, 45,
    48, 56, 58, 79, 88, 99, 114
high blood pressure, 19, 20
hip-hop, 113, 114
Honduras, 11, 12, 13, 21, 25,
    29, 30, 39, 41, 43, 47, 50, 64,
    73, 77, 78, 88, 90, 93, 101,
    108, 110, 111
hot spring, 42, 105, 124
huts, 42, 87
hybrid, 27, 28, 104

hybrids, 27, 30, 64, 65, 93
hypothyroidism, 74

Ilanga, 25
immune system, 27, 65, 93,
    95, 104, 120, 138
impotence, 13, 48, 75, 114
independence, 66, 67, 101,
    123, 125
iron, 53, 55, 77, 85, 100, 134,
    142, 144, 145, 146, 147, 148

Jack LaLanne, 127
Jethro Kloss, 139

Key West, 123

La Ceiba, 11, 12, 41, 42, 73,
    112, 127
leaders, 86, 95, 101, 102, 103,
    104, 105, 107, 111
Lisa "Left Eye" Lopes, 50,
    113

Mama Hay, 40, 100, 108, 109,
    110, 123, 124, 125, 126
Marcus Garvey, 124, 125
Matun, 38, 40, 42, 43, 53, 112
Max Robinson, 119
meat, 18, 61, 77, 78, 89, 90,
    110, 127
Medicinal Herbs, 152
Melvin Lindsey, 119

merchant seaman, 41, 111,
    114
Michael Jackson, 50, 121
milk, 31, 66, 79, 138, 139, 155,
    159, 161, 162, 164, 196
mucous, 16, 31, 37, 77, 78, 79
mushrooms, 31, 95, 137, 178,
    179, 180, 182, 188, 189

natural, 12, 13, 26, 27, 28, 29,
    38, 43, 55, 56, 63, 64, 65, 66,
    69, 73, 77, 93, 94, 97, 100,
    104, 109, 110, 114, 120, 125,
    134, 137, 138, 139, 142, 151,
    155, 196
nature, 9, 42, 45, 56, 65, 66,
    67, 107
navy bean, 76
Negro, 17, 124
Nigeria, 90
nutrition, 29, 49, 111, 128
nutritionist, 28, 65, 77, 91,
    116

obesity, 13, 75
organic, 13, 29, 55, 138, 185

Paavo Airola, 65
pH, 28, 31, 56, 105, 138
plant, 11, 27, 65, 66, 73, 99,
    100, 110, 123, 145, 146, 147

rice, 16, 17, 31, 48, 54, 67, 71,
    77, 100, 110, 189

sea moss elixir, 53
selective breeding, 27
Sinusitis, 31
soul food, 17
South Africa, 106
South Carolina, 16, 18, 94
southern cooking, 16, 18
Spanish, 26, 41, 42, 63, 138,
   142, 143, 145, 146, 148
spelt, 92
spelt harvesting, 93
starch, 16, 19, 48, 64, 65, 71,
   73, 74, 76, 77, 78, 87, 89,
   131, 134, 141, 149

*The Cure: The Autobiography
   of Dr. Sebi "Mama Hay,* 123
The Fig Tree, 38
thermal water, 43, 55

tropics, 43, 47, 143, 144

unnatural, 56, 64, 79, 100
Usha Research Institute, 77,
   124, 125
Usha Village, 12, 29, 42, 43,
   47, 53, 55, 57, 66, 86, 87, 93,
   101, 103, 112, 113, 123, 124

vegetarian, 12, 26, 29, 30, 134,
   135, 139

Washington, DC, 14, 16, 18,
   21, 25, 40, 48, 50, 113, 118,
   119, 120
World Health Organization,
   51, 87, 201

Zimbabwe, 50, 74, 105, 106